A Colour Atlas of
ENDOCRINOLOGY
Second Edition

R. HALL, CBE, BSc, MD, FRCP
Professor of Medicine,
University of Wales College of Medicine

D. C. EVERED, BSc, MD, FRCP, FIBiol
Second Secretary,
Medical Research Council

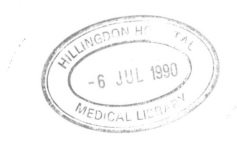
Wolfe Medical Publications Ltd

Copyright © R. Hall, D. C. Evered, 1990
Published by Wolfe Medical Publications Ltd, 1990
Printed by Royal Smeets Offset, Weert, Netherlands
ISBN 0 7234 1560 9

A CIP catalogue record for this book is available from the
British Library.

This book is one of the titles in the series of Wolfe Medical
Atlases, a series that brings together the world's largest
systematic published collection of diagnostic colour
photographs. For a full list of Atlases in the series, plus
forthcoming titles and details of our surgical, dental and
veterinary Atlases, please write to Wolfe Medical
Publications Ltd, 2-16 Torrington Place, London
WC1E 7LT, England.

Contents

Introduction

The objective of this Atlas is to illustrate the clinical features of endocrine disease and the many related disorders which are commonly referred to endocrine clinics.

Endocrinology is a specialty with a large but variable visual content. Some topics, including the most prevalent endocrine disorders, such as diabetes mellitus and thyroid, adrenal and pituitary diseases have many features which can be clearly illustrated, whereas others, including aldosteronism and phaeochromocytoma have very few visual features that can be demonstrated by clinical photographs. We have, therefore, overcome this problem by introducing line diagrams to accompany the photographs and the text.

The emphasis of this book is on clinical presentation, diagnosis and the improvements which may be seen with treatment. This new edition has been very substantially revised. The text has been extensively rewritten and now provides much fuller coverage of the clinical features of endocrine and related disorders than the first edition. The number of illustrations has been increased from 500 to nearly 1,000, and over 70 per cent of these are entirely new. It is effectively a new book.

It is intended that this volume will be of practical value for all those concerned in the management of patients with endocrine diseases. It will also provide an invaluable guide for undergraduates and postgraduates preparing for graduation and for higher qualifications in medicine: clinical examinations frequently include endocrine cases.

R. Hall, D. C. Evered

Acknowledgements

The authors gratefully acknowledge the generosity of their many colleagues, listed below, who have allowed them to reproduce slides from their collections.

Dr D. Ackery, MB, MSc, FRCR
Consultant in Nuclear Medicine,
Southampton General Hospital,
Southampton SO9 4XY.

Dr D. Adams, MDS, BSc, PhD *Reader in Oral Biology,*
Department of Basic Dental Science,
Dental School,
Cardiff.

Dr J. Adams, MD
Reproductive Endocrine Unit,
Massachusetts General Hospital,
Boston,
Massachusetts 02114.

Dr G. Anderson, MD, FRCP
Consultant Physician
Newport Chest Clinic,
129 Stow Hill,
Newport, Gwent NP9 4GA.

Professor John Anderson, MB, BS, FRCP, FRCOG
Regional Postgraduate Dean and Professor of Medical Education,
University of Newcastle upon Tyne,
Regional Postgraduate Institute for Medicine and Dentistry,
11 Framlington Place,
Newcastle upon Tyne NE2 4AB.

Dr C. N. Armstrong, MD, FRCP
Consulting Physician
Royal Victoria Infirmary
Newcastle upon Tyne NE1 4LP.

Dr J. Bagg, BDS, PhD, FDS, RCS (Ed.)
Lecturer in Oral Pathology,
Department of Oral Medicine,
Oral Pathology and Oral Surgery,
Dental School,
Cardiff.

Dr D. Bates, MA, MB, BChir, FRCP
Senior Lecturer in Neurology,
Department of Neurology,
University of Newcastle upon Tyne
NE1 4LP.

Sir Richard Bayliss, KCVO, MD, FRCP
Flat 7
61 Onslow Square,
London SW7 3LS.

L. Beck, FRCS, FCOphth
Consultant Ophthalmologist,
Department of Ophthalmology,
University Hospital of Wales,
Cardiff CF4 4XW.

K. Bellamy, ARPS, AIMBI
Senior Medical Photographer in Charge,
Cardiff Royal Infirmary,
Newport Road,
Cardiff.

Professor G. M. Besser, MD, FRCP
Department of Endocrinology,
Medical College of St Bartholomew's Hospital,
King George V Building,
West Smithfield,
London EC1A 7BE.

Professor S. R. Bloom, MA, MD, DSc, FRCP
Professor of Endocrinology,
Department of Medicine,
Hammersmith Hospital,
London W12 0HS.

Dr C. G. D. Brook, MD, FRCP
Consultant Paediatrician,
The Middlesex Hospital,
Mortimer Street,
London W1N 8AA.

Dr F. Clark, MB, BS, FRCP
Consultant Physician and Senior Lecturer in Medicine,
Freeman Hospital,
Newcastle upon Tyne NE7 7DN.

Professor A. S. Compston, FRCP, PhD
Professor of Neurology,
University of Cambridge School of Clinical Medicine.
Addenbrooke's Hospital,
Hills Road,
Cambridge.

Dr J. Compston, MD, FRCP
Senior Lecturer/Honorary Consultant,
Department of Pathology,
University of Wales College of Medicine,
Heath Park,
Cardiff CF4 4XN.

Professor V. A. Cowie, MD, PhD, FRCPsych, DPM
lately Professor of Mental Handicap,
Academic Unit of Mental Handicap,
Ely Hospital,
University of Wales College of Medicine,
Cardiff.

Professor A. L. Crombie, MB, ChB, FRCS (Ed.), FCOphth
Professor of Ophthalmology and Associate Dean of the Medical School,
University of Newcastle upon Tyne,
Framlington Place,
Newcastle upon Tyne NE2 4HH.

Dr A. Davies, MRCP
Morriston Hospital,
Swansea.

J. Dunlop,
Senior Medical Photographer,
University Hospital of Wales,
Heath Park,
Cardiff CF4 4XN.

J. R. G. Edwards, FRCS
former Consultant Plastic Surgeon,
Royal Victoria Infirmary,
Newcastle upon Tyne NE1 4LP.

Dr A. W. Finlay, MB, BS, MRCP, LRCP
Senior Lecturer in Dermatology,
Department of Medicine,
University of Wales College of Medicine,
Heath Park,
Cardiff CF4 4XN.

Dr J. C. Forfar, MD, PhD, FRCPE
Consultant Cardiologist,
John Radcliffe Hospital,
Oxford OX3 9DU.

Dr H. Gharib, MD, FACP
Associate Professor of Medicine
Mayo Medical School,
Rochester, Minnesota,
USA.

Dr D. B. Grant, MD, FRCP, DCH
Consultant Paediatric
Endocrinologist,
The Hospital for Sick Children,
Great Ormond Street,
London WC1N 3JH.

Dr I. H. Gravelle, BSc, MB, ChB,
FRCPE, FRCR
Senior Consultant Radiologist,
University Hospital of Wales,
Heath Park,
Cardiff CF4 4XN.

Professor O. P. Gray, MB, ChB,
FRCP, DCH
Head of Child Health,
University of Wales College of
Medicine,
Heath Park,
Cardiff CF4 4XN.

P. J. Gregory, BSc, MSc
Principal Cytogeneticist,
Cytogenetics Unit for Wales,
Institute of Medical Genetics,
University Hospital of Wales,
Heath Park,
Cardiff CF4 4XN.

Dr P. M. Hacking, MA, MD, FRCR
Consultant Radiologist,
Department of Radiology,
The Royal Victoria Infirmary and
University of Newcastle upon Tyne,
Queen Victoria Road,
Newcastle upon Tyne NE1 4LP.

J. W. Haggith, BSc, CPhys, FInstP,
FIPSM
Top Grade Physicist,
Regional Medical Physics
Department,
Newcastle General Hospital,
Westgate Road,
Newcastle upon Tyne NE4 6BE.

Dr M. Hall, MB, FRCP
Consultant Physician,
Caerphilly District Miners Hospital,
and Consultant Rheumatologist,
University Hospital of Wales,
Heath Park,
Cardiff CF4 4XN.

Professor T. M. Hayes, MB, ChB,
FRCP
Director and Dean of Postgraduate
Studies,
University of Wales College of
Medicine,
Heath Park,
Cardiff CF4 4XN.

Dr M. W. J. Hayward, FRCS, FRCR
Senior Lecturer in Diagnostic
Radiology,
University of Wales College of
Medicine,
Heath Park,
Cardiff CF4 4XN.

Professor B. M. Hibbard, MD, PhD,
FRCOG
Professor & Head of Department of
Obstetrics & Gynaecology,
University of Wales College of
Medicine,
Heath Park,
Cardiff CF4 4XN.

Dr G. Holti, MD, FRCP
Honorary Consultant Dermatologist,
Newcastle Health Authority,
211 Middle Drive,
Ponteland,
Newcastle upon Tyne NE20 9LU.

Dr M. D. Hourihan, MB, BCh, FRCR
Consultant Neuroradiologist,
University Hospital of Wales,
Heath Park,
Cardiff CF4 4XN.

Dr P. Hudgson, FRCP, FRACP
Consultant and Senior Lecturer,
Clinical Director (Adult
Neuromuscular Diseases Clinic),
Regional Neurological Centre,
Newcastle General Hospital,
Newcastle upon Tyne NE4 6BE.

A. Hughes, BSc
Senior Medical Photographer,
University Hospital of Wales,
Heath Park,
Cardiff CF4 4XN.

Dr I. A. Hughes, MD, FRCP, FRCP (C)
Reader in Child Health,
University of Wales College of
Medicine, Cardiff, and
Professor of Paediatrics – Elect,
University of Cambridge Clinical
School,
Department of Paediatrics,
Level 8, Addenbrooke's Hospital,
Hills Road,
Cambridge CB2 2QQ.

Dr F. Ive, MB, FRCP
Consultant Dermatologist,
Dryburn Hospital,
Durham.

Professor H. S. Jacobs, MD, FRCP
Professor of Reproductive
Endocrinology,
University College and Middlesex
School of Medicine,
Cobbold Laboratories,
Middlesex Hospital,
Mortimer Street,
London W1N 8AA.

Professor O. F. W. James, MA, FRCP
Professor of Geriatric Medicine,
University of Newcastle upon Tyne,
Framlington Place,
Newcastle upon Tyne NE2 4HH.

Dr E. M. Jepson, MD, FRCP
Consultant Physician,
Parkside,
Central Middlesex Hospital,
Acton Lane,
London NW1 7NS.

Professor I. D. A. Johnston, MCh,
FRCS,
FACS (Hon)
Professor and Head of Department of
Surgery,
University of Newcastle upon Tyne,
Department of Surgery,
The Medical School,
Newcastle upon Tyne NE2 4HH.

Professor G. F. Joplin, PhD, FRCP
Professor of Clinical Endocrinology
and Consultant Physician,
Royal Postgraduate Medical School,
Du Cane Road,
London W12 0NN.

Professor P. Kendall-Taylor, DCH,
MD, FRCP
Professor of Endocrinology and
Consultant Physician,
Department of Medicine,
Medical School,
University of Newcastle upon Tyne,
NE2 4HH.

Professor D. N. S. Kerr, MD, FRCP
Dean,
Royal Postgraduate Medical School,
Hammersmith Hospital,
Du Cane Road,
London W12 0HS.

Professor M. Laurence, MA, MB, ChB, DSc, FRCP (Ed.), FRCPath
Consultant Clinical Geneticist,
Institute of Medical Genetics,
University of Wales College of Medicine,
Heath Park,
Cardiff CF4 4XN.

Dr J. H. Lazarus, MA, MD, FRCP
Senior Lecturer,
Department of Medicine,
University of Wales College of Medicine,
Heath Park,
Cardiff CF4 4XN.

Dr J. M. Marks, DM, FRCP
Senior Lecturer in Dermatology,
University of Newcastle upon Tyne,
and Honorary Consultant Dermatologist,
Newcastle Hospitals,
University Department of Dermatology,
Royal Victoria Infirmary,
Newcastle upon Tyne NE1 4LP.

Professor R. Marks, FRCP, FRCPath
Professor of Dermatology,
University of Wales College of Medicine,
Heath Park,
Cardiff CF4 4XN.

B. Marshall, SRN
Senior Medical Photographer,
Department of Medical Illustration,
University of Wales College of Medicine,
Heath Park,
Cardiff CF4 4XN.

Professor R. Marshall, PhD, Hon. FRPS, Hon. FBIPP, AIMBI
Director of Medical Illustration,
University of Wales College of Medicine,
Heath Park,
Cardiff CF4 4XN.

Professor A. M. McGregor, MA, MD, FRCP
Professor of Medicine,
Department of Medicine,
King's College Hospital Medical School,
Denmark Hill,
London SE5 8RX.

Professor B. McKibbin, MS, MD, FRCS
Professor of Traumatic and Orthopaedic Surgery,
University of Wales College of Medicine,
Heath Park,
Cardiff CF4 4XN.

L. Mir, SRN, SCN
Sister,
Department of Medicine,
University Hospital of Wales,
Heath Park,
Cardiff CF4 4XN.

Dr M. A. Mir, DCH, FRCP
Senior Lecturer,
Department of Medicine,
University of Wales College of Medicine,
Heath Park,
Cardiff CF4 4XN.

Professor J. L. H. O'Riordan, DM, FRCP
Professor of Metabolic Medicine,
The Middlesex Hospital,
London W1 8AA.

Dr D. R. Owens, MD
Senior Lecturer,
Diabetes Research Unit,
Department of Medicine,
University of Wales College of Medicine,
Heath Park,
Cardiff CF4 4XN.

Dr M. D. Page, MRCP
Honorary Registrar and Wellcome Trust Medical Graduate Fellow,
Department of Medicine,
University of Wales College of Medicine,
Heath Park,
Cardiff CF4 4XN.

Professor M. Parkin, MD, FRCP
Professor of Clinical Paediatrics,
Department of Child Health,
The Medical School,
University of Newcastle upon Tyne NE2 4HH.

Dr W. J. Penny, MD, FRCP
Consultant Cardiologist,
Department of Cardiology,
University Hospital of Wales,
Heath Park,
Cardiff CF4 4XN.

Professor P. O. D. Pharoah, MD, MSc, FFCM
Professor of Community Medicine,
University of Liverpool,
PO Box 147,
Liverpool L69 3BX.

Dr R. M. Pope, MB, BCh, MRCP
MRC Training Fellow,
Department of Medicine,
King's College Hospital Medical School,
Denmark Hill,
London SE5 8RX.

Dr W. H. Price, FRCP (Ed.)
Physician,
Department of Medicine,
Western General Hospital,
Edinburgh EH4 2XU.

Dr J. M. Rao, MRCPsych, DPM
Consultant Psychiatrist,
Ely Hospital,
Cowbridge Road West,
Cardiff.

Dr J. A. E. Rees, BSc, MD, MRCP
Wellcome Senior Research Fellow in Clinical Science and Senior Lecturer,
Department of Medicine,
University of Wales College of Medicine,
Heath Park,
Cardiff CF4 4XN.

Professor M. F. Scanlon, BSc, MD, FRCP
Professor of Endocrinology,
Department of Medicine,
University of Wales College of Medicine,
Heath Park,
Cardiff CF4 4XN.

Dr D. G. Seymour, BSc, MB, ChB, MRCP
Senior Lecturer,
Department of Geriatric Medicine,
University of Wales College of Medicine,
Heath Park,
Cardiff CF4 4XN.

A. Shaw
Medical Artist,
Department of Medical Illustration,
University of Wales College of Medicine,
Heath Park,
Cardiff CF4 4XN.

Professor D. A. Shaw, MB, ChB,
FRCP, FRCP (Ed.)
*Dean and Professor of Clinical
Neurology,
The Medical School,
University of Newcastle upon Tyne,
Framlington Place,
Newcastle upon Tyne NE2 4HH.*

R. Skinner, ABIPP
*Senior Medical Photographer,
Department of Medical Illustration,
University of Wales College of
Medicine,
Heath Park,
Cardiff CF4 4XN.*

Dr P. M. Smith, MD, FRCP
*Consultant Physician and
Gastroenterologist,
University Hospital of Wales
and Llandough Hospital,
Cardiff.*

Professor R. E. Steiner, CBE, MD,
FRCP, FRCS, FRCR
*Professor of Radiology,
Hammersmith Hospital,
Du Cane Road,
London W12 0HS.*

D. Tacchi, MD, FRCOG
*Consultant Obstetrician and
Gynaecologist,
Honorary Lecturer,
University Department of Obstetrics
and Gynaecology,
Princess Mary Maternity Hospital,
Great North Road,
Newcastle upon Tyne.*

Professor G. Teasdale, MB, FRCSE,
MRCP
*Department of Neurosurgery,
University of Glasgow,
Southern General Hospital,
Glasgow G51 4TF.*

Dr J. P. Thomas, MD, FRCP
*Consultant Physician,
Department of Medicine,
Ward B7
University Hospital of Wales,
Heath Park,
Cardiff CF4 4XN.*

Dr W. van't Hoff, MB, FRCP
*Formerly Consultant Physician,
Department of Endocrinology,
North Staffs Hospital Centre,
Stoke on Trent,
Staffs.*

M. H. Wheeler, MD, FRCS
*Consultant Surgeon,
Department of Surgery,
University Hospital of Wales,
Heath Park,
Cardiff CF4 4XN.*

Dr R. Wilkinson, MD, FRCP
*Reader in Medicine,
University of Newcastle upon Tyne,
and Freeman Hospital,
Newcastle upon Tyne NE7 7DN.*

Dr J. D. Williams, MD, MRCP
*Director of KRUF Institute of Renal
Disease,
Department of Medicine,
University of Wales College of
Medicine,
Cardiff Royal Infirmary,
Newport Road,
Cardiff.*

Professor V. Wright, MD, FRCP
*Professor of Rheumatology,
University of Leeds,
Leeds LS2 9JT.*

Chapter 1
Hypothalamus and pituitary

Introduction

The hypothalamus lies at the base of the brain and is connected to the pituitary by the pituitary stalk. Its major role is as a centre integrating and coordinating pituitary function, thermostasis, water, mineral and calorie balance, and sexual and reproductive activity. There are no neural connections between the hypothalamus and the anterior pituitary, and the hypothalamus influences and regulates pituitary function through the hypothalamo–hypophyseal portal system. The hypothalamus secretes a number of regulatory factors (releasing or inhibiting hormones) — see Table 1.

Table 1.

Hypothalamic hormones	Pituitary hormones
Thyrotrophin releasing hormone (TRH)	Thyrotrophin (TSH)
	Prolactin
Gonadotrophin releasing hormone (GnRH)	Luteinising hormone (LH)
	Follicle stimulating hormone (FSH)
Somatostatin	Growth hormone (GH)
Growth hormone releasing hormone (GHRH)	
Corticotrophin releasing hormone (CRH)	Corticotrophin (ACTH)
Dopamine	Prolactin

A number of other weak interactions occur between the hypothalamic and the pituitary hormones, but these appear to be of little physiological significance. Somatostatin is also secreted by many tissues which are not of neural origin and exerts a local paracrine action.

The posterior pituitary is not a discrete endocrine gland but merely the distal part of an endocrine neurosecretory system, which also includes various hypothalamic areas. The antidiuretic hormone is secreted by the supraoptic and paraventricular nuclei and passes down the neurohypophyseal tract linked with neurophysin to be stored in the posterior lobe and then secreted into the general circulation.

Diseases of the hypothalamus and pituitary

Disturbances of secretion of the hypothalamic regulatory hormones

Deficient production of the hypothalamic hormones commonly results from tumours (particularly craniopharyngiomas, chromophobe adenomas and secondary carcinomas), granulomatous disorders (histiocytosis X, tuberculosis and sarcoidosis) or trauma. The deficiencies may lead to a variety of pituitary hormone deficits but, in general, luteinising hormone and growth hormone production are affected early, often in combination with hyperprolactinaemia, and the secretion of the other pituitary hormones is often conserved until later in the course of the disease. Hypothalamic disorders are frequently associated with diabetes insipidus, and visual field defects may occur particularly if a hypothalamic tumour is present. Other disturbances of hypothalamic function may occur, including disturbances of appetite and thirst, altered thermostasis and abnormal sleep patterns. The major clinical features of failure of secretion of the hypothalamic hormones, however, result from the secondary failure of the pituitary hormones and these disorders will, therefore, be considered together as disturbances of hypothalamic–pituitary function.

Overproduction of certain hypothalamic hormones may be responsible for certain conditions, but these are rare. Ectopic production of corticotrophin releasing hormone has been reported as a rare cause of Cushing's disease resulting from bilateral adrenal hyperplasia, and production of growth hormone releasing hormone from a peripheral carcinoid tumour may very rarely cause acromegaly. Early production of gonadotrophin releasing hormone may be responsible for the precocious puberty seen in polyostotic fibrous dysplasia (Albright's syndrome). These conditions are dealt with in the section on hypothalamic–pituitary disease, and also in Chapters 5 and 9.

Clinical features of hypothalamic–pituitary disease

The six common presentations of hypothalamic–pituitary disease are as follows:

- Partial or complete failure of pituitary hormone production (**1**)
- Acromegaly (**2** and **3**) or gigantism
- Cushing's syndrome (**4**)
- Galactorrhoea (**5**)

- Diabetes insipidus
- Pituitary or hypothalamic tumour — which may be asymptomatic, or associated with any of the endocrine problems listed above, or the cause of pressure effects on adjacent structures. Illustration **6** shows an enlarged pituitary fossa on a lateral skull radiograph in close-up.

1

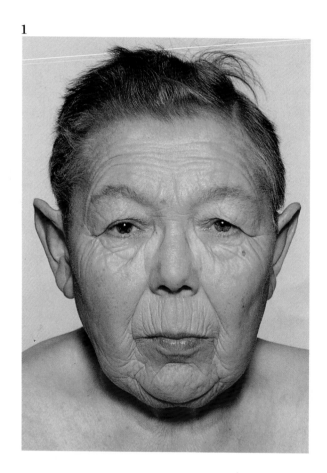

2

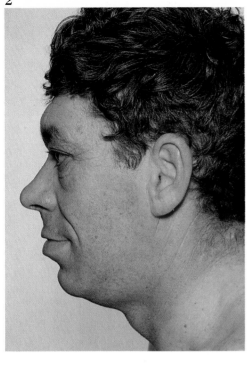

3

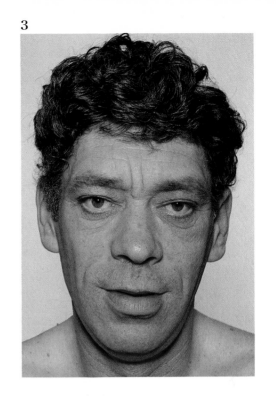

4

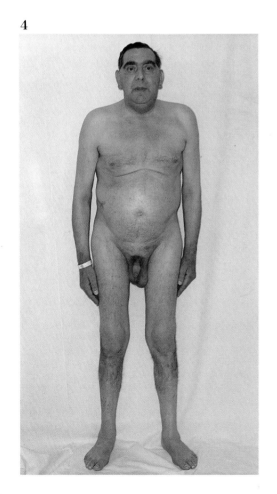

5

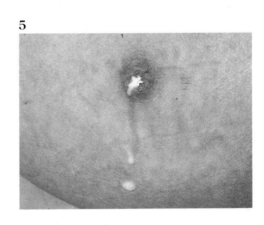

6

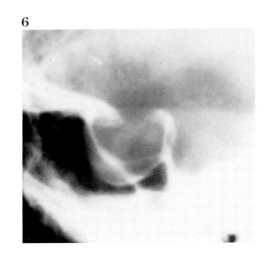

Pituitary failure

Pituitary failure commonly results from an adenoma, infarction or trauma (or more rarely from a secondary neoplasm, chronic infection, granuloma or lipoidosis). The major clinical features reflect the degree of failure, the pattern of hormonal deficiency and the local effects of the underlying pathology and are shown in **7**. Partial hypopituitarism is much commoner than panhypopituitarism.

7

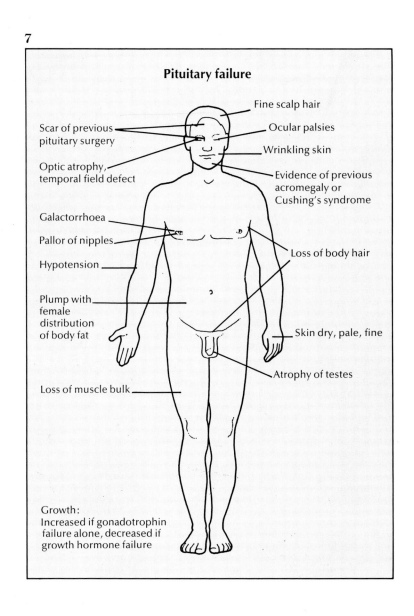

Pituitary failure

Fine scalp hair

Scar of previous pituitary surgery

Ocular palsies

Wrinkling skin

Optic atrophy, temporal field defect

Evidence of previous acromegaly or Cushing's syndrome

Galactorrhoea

Pallor of nipples

Hypotension

Loss of body hair

Plump with female distribution of body fat

Skin dry, pale, fine

Atrophy of testes

Loss of muscle bulk

Growth:
Increased if gonadotrophin failure alone, decreased if growth hormone failure

Gonadotrophin failure occurs early in pituitary disease and thus impotence in the male and amenorrhoea in the female are common early symptoms. The clinical features include fine wrinkling of the skin round the mouth (**8** and **9**), loss of facial (**10**) and body hair (**11** and **12**), atrophy of the genitalia (**13**) in both sexes and sometimes loss of breast tissue in the female.

8

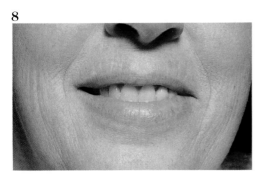

9

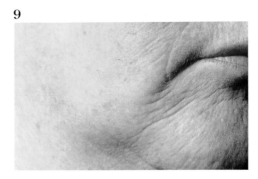

10

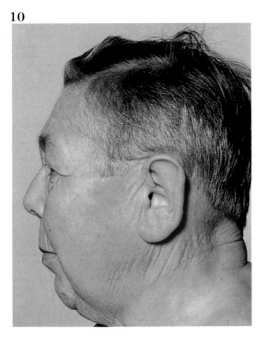

11

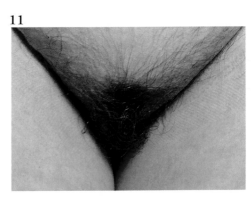

12

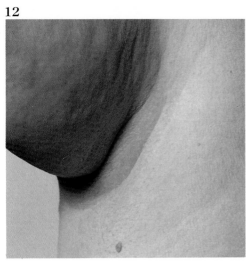

13

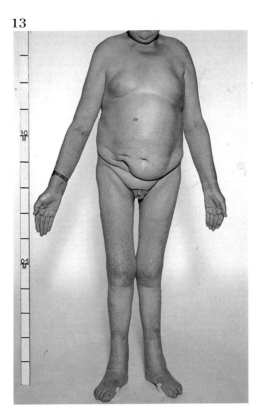

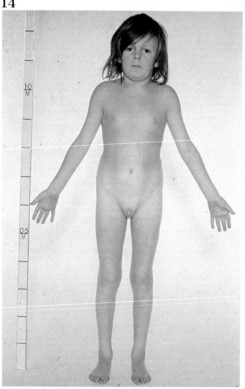

Gonadotrophin failure in childhood leads to failure of puberty (**14**), although this must be distinguished from constitutional delay of puberty which may mimic pituitary failure (**15** — see also Chapter 5), and if growth hormone is normal, excessive linear growth as the epiphyses fuse late. The presence of gonadotrophin failure can be finally established only by the lack of pubertal development over a period of time. Low or normal gonadotrophin levels, in association with the clinical features described above, are not alone sufficient evidence to confirm pituitary gonadotrophin failure. Isolated gonadotrophin deficiency associated with anosmia is seen in Kallmann's syndrome (**16**).

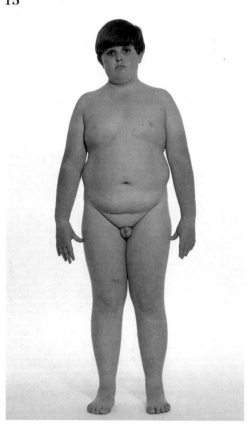

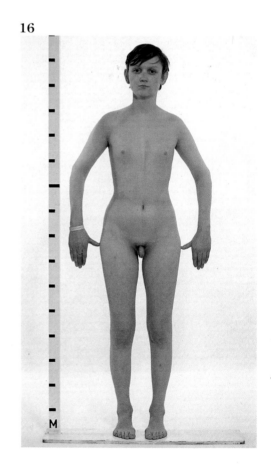

Growth hormone deficiency in children leads to dwarfism and delayed skeletal and dental development. Illustration **17** shows a 10-year-old child with a height of 1.15m (the third centile for a child of this age is 1.24m). Plumpness is common and fine wrinkling of the skin may be seen in the adult even in the absence of gonadotrophin deficiency. Growth hormone deficiency can be confirmed by the finding of low growth hormone levels which do not rise in response to hypoglycaemia (in an insulin sensitivity test) or arginine. Assessing the response to exercise or to meat extract, as has been recommended in the past, are less satisfactory alternatives for testing endogenous growth hormone secretion. Disorders of growth will be considered further in Chapter 2.

17

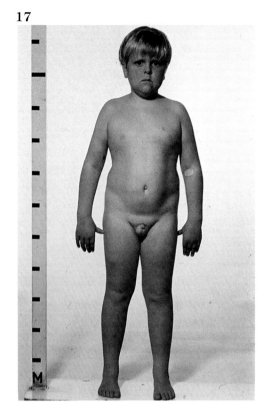

Thyrotrophin (TSH) deficiency will give rise to features similar to those seen in primary hypothyroidism. These include dryness of the skin (**18**), although the skin does not usually become so coarse as in primary thyroid failure. Thyrotrophin deficiency may contribute to growth retardation in children (**19**). It may be difficult to recognise clinically and the diagnosis is confirmed by finding low thyroid hormone levels without elevation of thyrotrophin (although minor elevation of TSH may be seen).

18

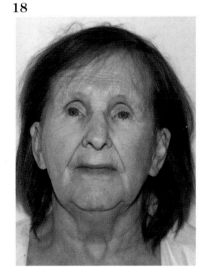

19

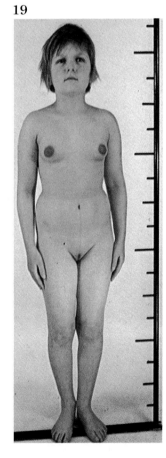

Corticotrophin (ACTH) deficiency is generally slow in onset leading to weakness, nausea, hypoglycaemia and collapse and coma if severe. Corticotrophin deficiency may contribute to pallor of the skin (20). The diagnosis is confirmed by finding low cortisol levels which do not rise adequately in response to hypoglycaemia.

20

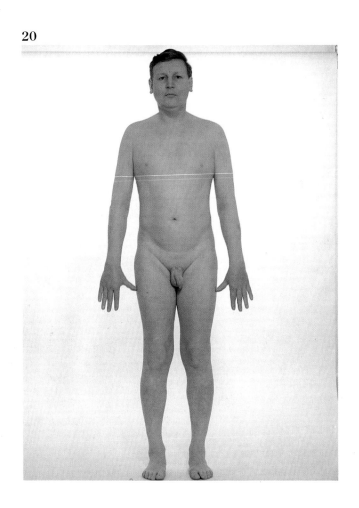

Acromegaly and gigantism

Acromegaly is the clinical condition which results from increased circulating growth hormone (GH) in the adult. Gigantism is its counterpart in childhood. The disease is usually insidious in onset and slow to progress. Illustrations **21** to **24** show a patient at the ages of 18, 25, 28 and 32 years.

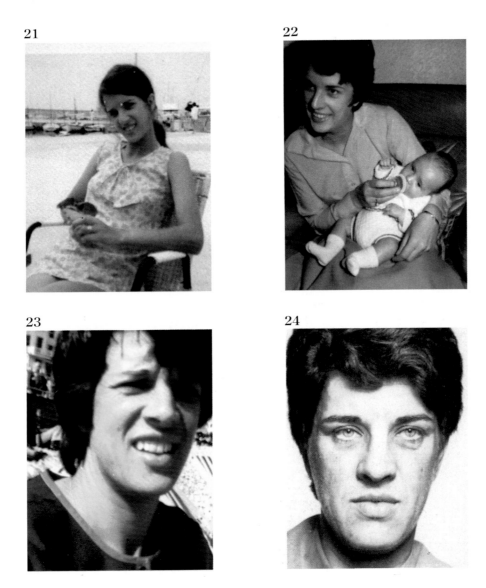

21

22

23

24

The presence of the disease is usually suspected from the **characteristic clinical features** (**25** and **26**) which vary in severity, and include thickening of soft tissues and skin, broadening of the nose, increased prominence of supraorbital and nuchal ridges, and prognathism (**27** to **30**), which may lead to malocclusion, and separation of the teeth (**31** and **32**).

26

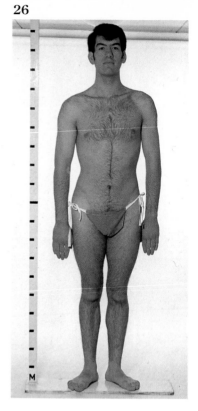

25

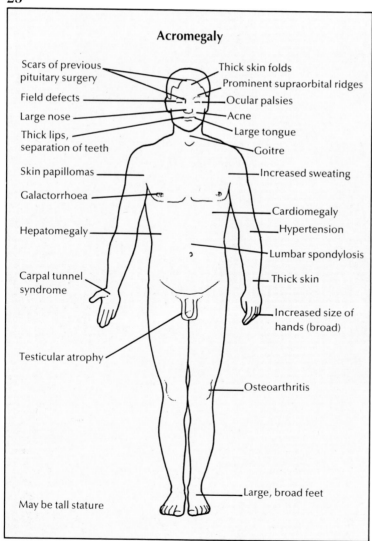

Acromegaly

Scars of previous pituitary surgery

Field defects

Large nose

Thick lips, separation of teeth

Skin papillomas

Galactorrhoea

Hepatomegaly

Carpal tunnel syndrome

Testicular atrophy

May be tall stature

Thick skin folds

Prominent supraorbital ridges

Ocular palsies

Acne

Large tongue

Goitre

Increased sweating

Cardiomegaly

Hypertension

Lumbar spondylosis

Thick skin

Increased size of hands (broad)

Osteoarthritis

Large, broad feet

27

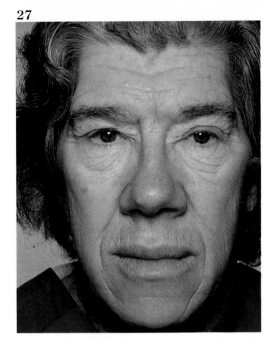

28

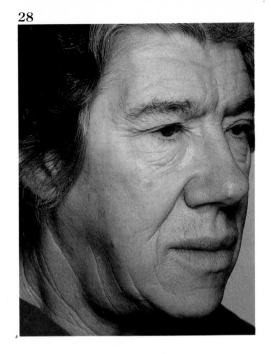

29

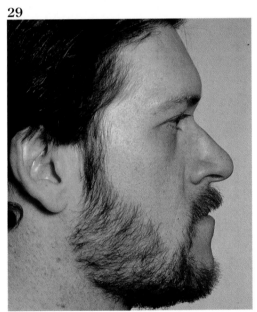

30

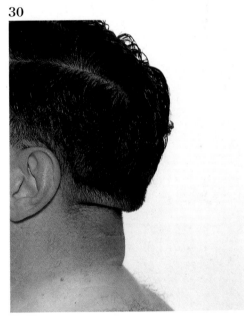

31

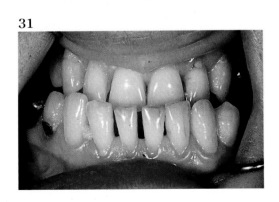

32

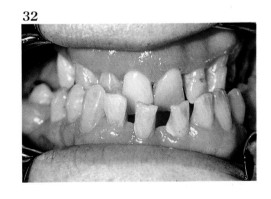

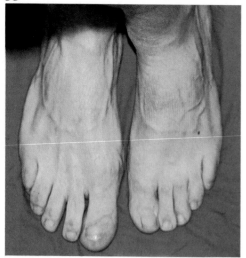

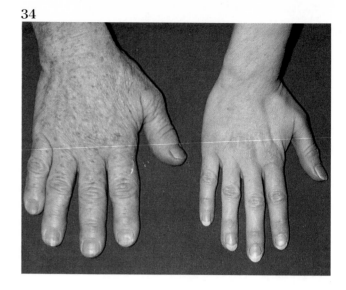

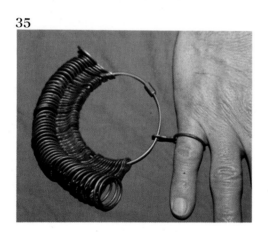

An increase in breadth of the hands and feet is obvious. Rings may become tight and the patient requires progressively larger sizes of shoes. **33** and **34** show an acromegalic foot and hand compared with those of a normal subject. Finger size can be assessed by the use of jeweller's rings (**35**). The general thickening of the soft tissues may cause compression of the median nerve at the wrist (carpal tunnel syndrome). The hand also provides a convenient site to assess skin thickness (**36**). The skinfold on the dorsum of the patient's hand can be compared with a skinfold on the dorsum of the examining hand.

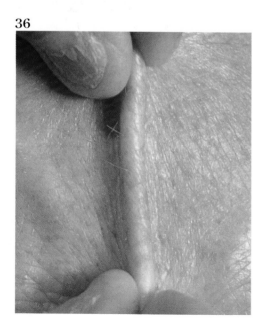

Other common clinical features include osteoarthrosis (**37**) characterised by an increased joint space resulting from an overgrowth of cartilage, increased laxity of ligaments (**38**), skin papillomata (**39**), acne (**40**), multiple lipomatosis (**41** and **42**) and cardiac failure (**43**). The cardiac failure may occur as a result of associated ischaemic heart disease, hypertension or cardiomyopathy.

37

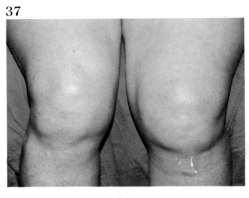

38

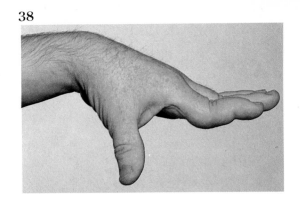

39

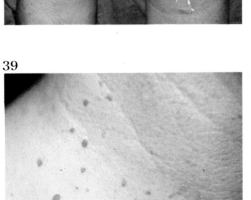

40

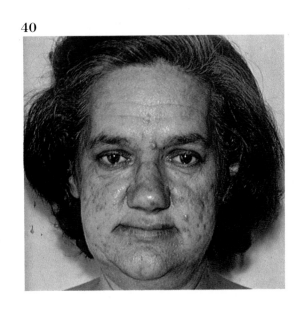

41

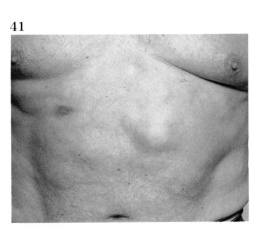

42

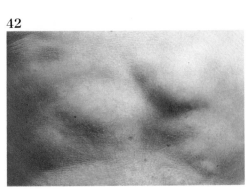

43

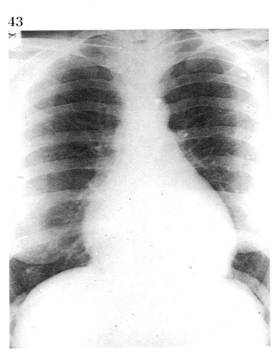

Cardiomegaly can also be demonstrated by echocardiography (**44** shows an acromegalic echocardiogram with septal hypertrophy and **45** a normal control).

Septal thickening can also be shown by a two-dimensional echocardiograph (**46** — acromegaly, **47** — normal).

44

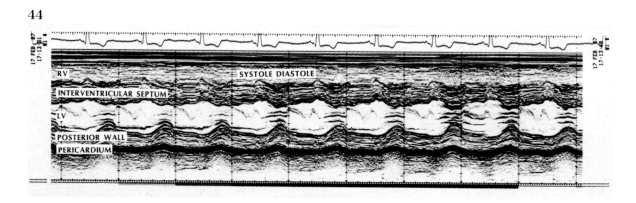

45

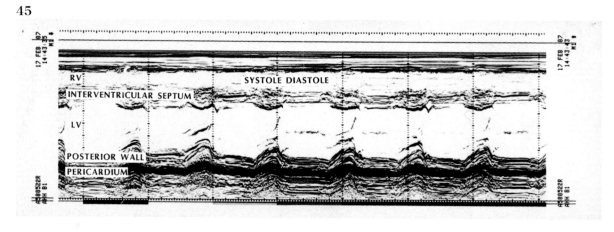

46

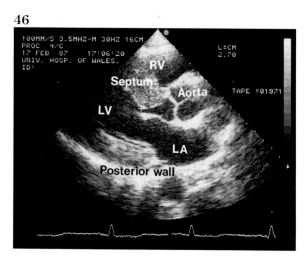

47

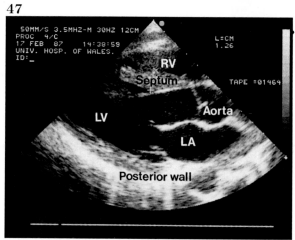

Enlargement of the tongue (**48**) and all the viscera is common. Hepatomegaly and splenomegaly may be found, and goitre (**49**) is present in 20 per cent of patients. Galactorrhoea is not uncommon (**50**) and varying degrees of pituitary failure (caused by expansion of the tumour) may be seen (see below).

48

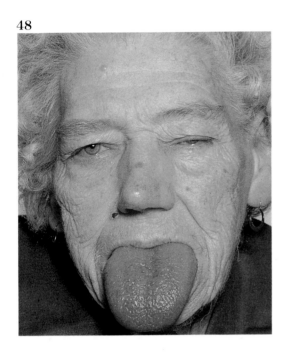

49

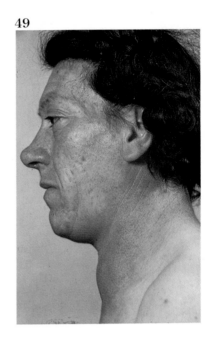

50

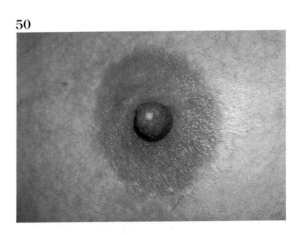

Visual field defects and other local effects of an expanding pituitary tumour may occur if the tumour extends outside the pituitary fossa (see below). The most common visual defects are a bitemporal upper quadrantic defect or a hemianopia. **51** shows field defects in acromegaly. Expansion of the pituitary fossa is seen on a lateral skull radiograph in 90 per cent of patients (**52**). Asymmetry of the floor is often the earliest radiological sign (**53**). The extent of the tumour can be clearly defined by CT scanning. **54** shows an adenoma (A) with a suprasellar extension (S), and **55** with suprasellar and lateral extensions.

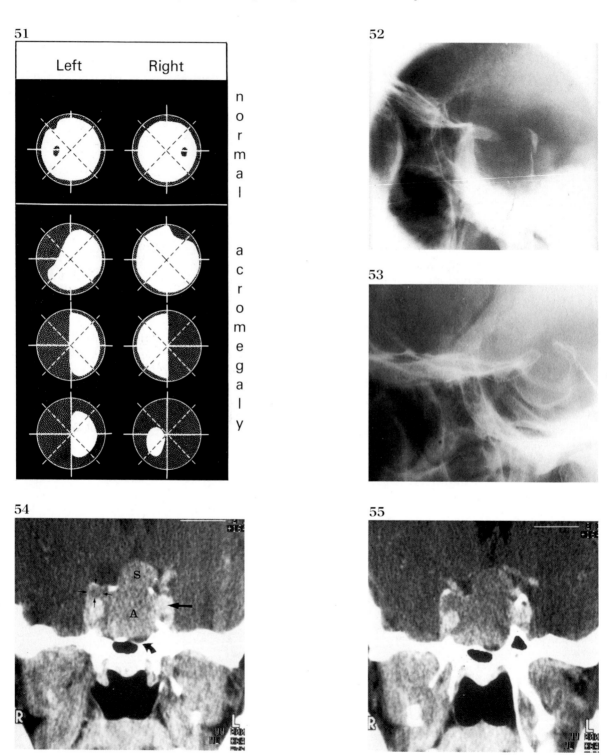

Increase in **heel pad thickness** (**56**) or skin thickness (**57**) may also be detected by appropriate radiological techniques.

56

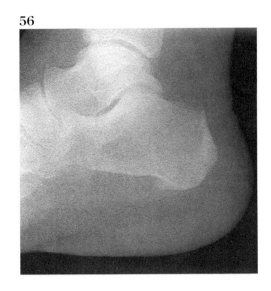

57

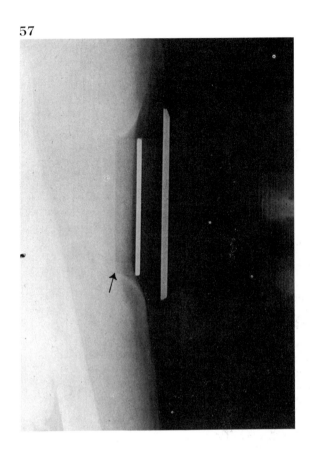

The diagnosis is confirmed by demonstrating an increase in growth hormone level which is not suppressed during a glucose tolerance test. Single estimations of GH are not reliable, as the hormone is normally secreted in a pulsatile manner in short bursts lasting one to two hours. The diagnosis should never be made on clinical grounds alone and biochemical confirmation should always be obtained. Some normal subjects with rugged features may have some of the characteristics of acromegaly (58), and some other conditions may mimic acromegaly — e.g. hypothyroidism with an increased soft tissue mass (59) and lipodystrophy (60). The patient's appearance may improve significantly after treatment (61). 62 and 63 show a profile and frontal view of another patient before treatment and two years after hypophysectomy. Further evaluation involves assessment of the size of the pituitary tumour, the degree to which other pituitary functions are disturbed and looking for complications.

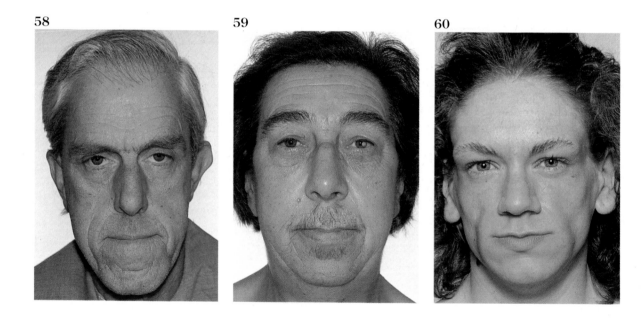

58   59   60

61

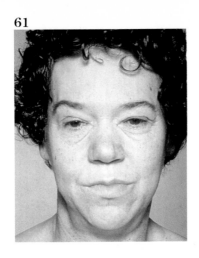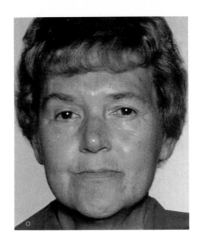

62

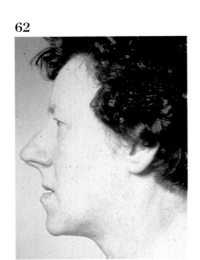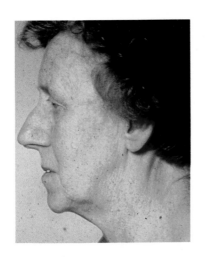

63

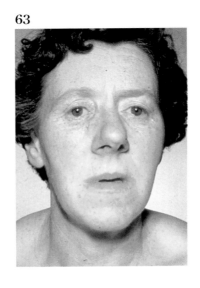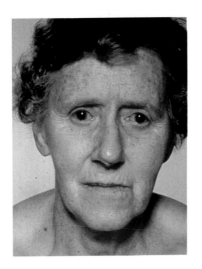

Gigantism results from increased GH levels before epiphyseal fusion. A marked increase in linear growth is evident. The soft tissue changes, though less obvious, are still present, probably because of the age of the patients and the shorter period between onset and diagnosis. **64** and **65** show a boy aged 16 years (1.95m in height) with features of gigantism and acromegaly. His final height, despite treatment, was 2.09m (**66** and **67** — same patient rephotographed at the age of 30 years). Causes of tall stature are described in greater detail in the chapter on growth and development (see pages 60 to 62).

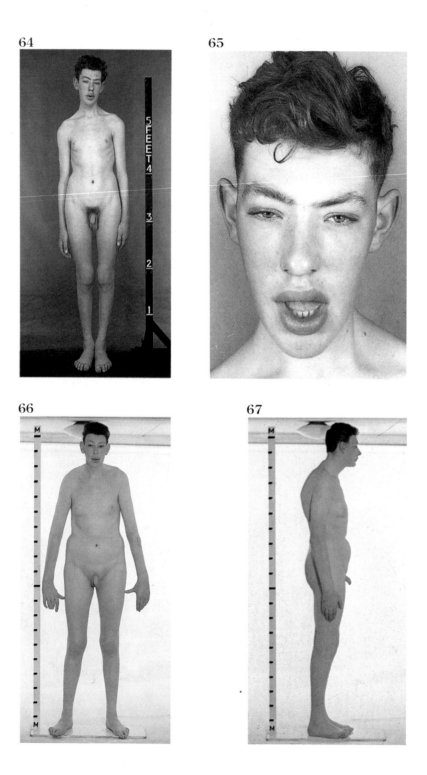

Cushing's syndrome

The term Cushing's syndrome describes those clinical disorders which result from an excess of circulating glucocorticoid. The term 'Cushing's disease' is currently used to describe patients in whom the syndrome results from an increase in pituitary ACTH production. Bilateral adrenal hyperplasia is found in this group and this is the commonest cause (approximately 90 per cent) of spontaneously occurring cases of Cushing's syndrome. The clinical features (**68**), other than the skin pigmentation resulting from high levels of ACTH, are almost exclusively related to the increase in adrenal steroid production and will therefore be considered in detail with other disorders of the adrenal (pages 118 to 130). **69** to **71** show a patient with Nelson's syndrome (pigmentation caused by increased ACTH production following bilateral adrenalectomy for Cushing's disease) — **69** and **70** were taken before removal of the adenoma, and **71** shows the patient after trans-sphenoidal hypophysectomy.

68

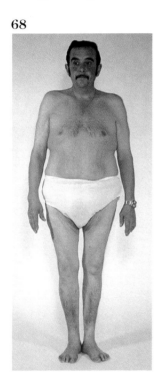

69

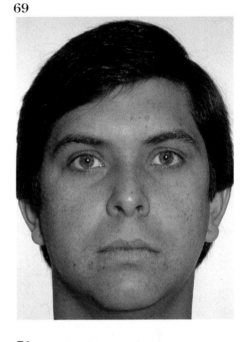

70

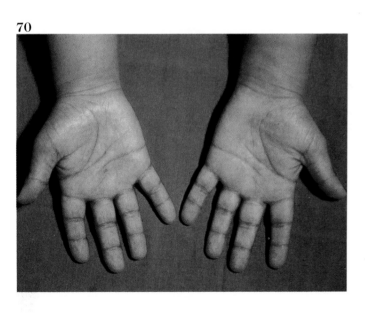

71

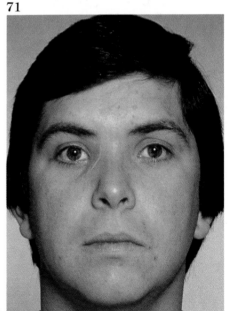

Galactorrhoea

Galactorrhoea is lactation in the absence of an appropriate physiological stimulus (**72** shows spontaneous galactorrhoea in a female and **73** on expression in a male). It may be unilateral or bilateral and may be evident only on expression. Occasionally thickening of the areolae and hyperplasia of Montgomery's tubercles may be seen. A serous or blood-stained discharge should always raise the possibility of an intrinsic breast lesion. It should be remembered that galactorrhoea may result from local lesions in the breast such as duct ectasia (**74**) and that some breast tumours, particularly intraduct lesions, cannot be detected on breast palpation. No specific signs are associated with galactorrhoea, but there may be signs which suggest the presence of a pituitary tumour (**75** shows a microadenoma on CT scan) or associated endocrine disease. Prolactinomas may undergo considerable expansion during pregnancy. The CT scans show a prolactinoma before (**76**) and during the third trimester of pregnancy (**77**). Prolonged hyperprolactinaemia causes hypogonadism and this possibility should be considered in patients presenting with infertility, amenorrhoea, impotence or other clinical features suggesting hypogonadism.

Table 2. Causes of galactorrhoea.

1. Hypothalamic or pituitary disease
   Hypothalamic or pituitary stalk disease
   Otherwise functionless adenomata
   Cushing's disease
   Acromegaly
2. Other endocrine disease
   Primary hypothyroidism
   Hyperthyroidism
3. Malignant disease
   Oestrogen-secreting tumours
   Prolactin-secreting tumours
4. Local disease or injury to the chest wall
5. Drugs
   Oral contraceptives
   Phenothiazines
   Tricyclic antidepressants
   Haloperidol
   Methyldopa
   Reserpine
   Metoclopramide
6. Chronic renal failure

72

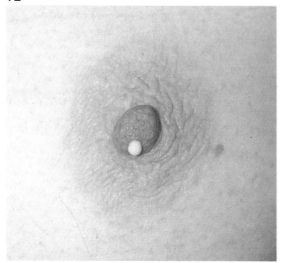

73

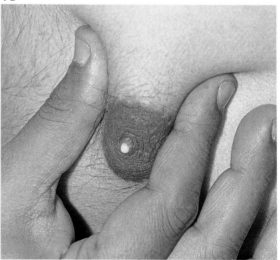

74

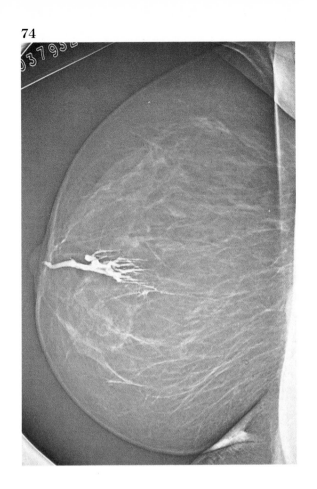

75

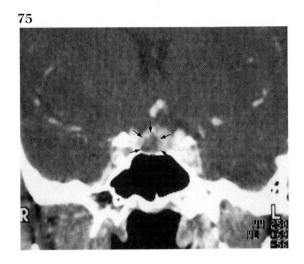

76

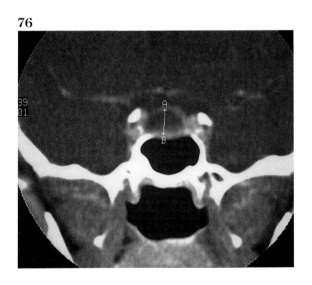

77

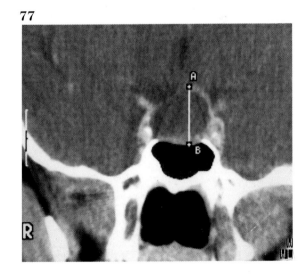

Diabetes insipidus

Diabetes insipidus results from ADH (vasopressin) deficiency (or rarely renal resistance to the hormone) and occurs uncommonly in patients with pituitary disease. Simple destruction of the posterior lobe or pituitary stalk at worst causes only transient diabetes insipidus, as ADH is able to escape directly into the general circulation from the axons of the hypothalamic neurones. A lesion has to be sufficiently large to produce considerable disturbance of the hypothalamus before diabetes insipidus occurs. The major organic lesions responsible for diabetes insipidus, therefore, are those which give rise to hypothalamic disease (see above). Diabetes insipidus is suspected in patients with a fluid intake and output greater than 2 litres in 24 hours.

Diabetes insipidus is frequently associated with a craniopharyngioma and may be accompanied by other hypothalamic disturbances — sleep disorders, hyperphagia or hypophagia, disturbed thermostasis, inappropriate reduction of thirst (leading to dehydration) and emotional behaviour. **78** shows a craniopharyngioma with calcification on a lateral skull radiograph.

Patients with polydipsia and polyuria may have primary polydipsia or primary polyuria (Table 3).

The **key investigations** that need to be done are demonstration of a high fluid throughput, estimation of serum osmolality and a fluid deprivation test. Diabetes insipidus and other causes of the primary polyuria syndromes are characterised by a high or high/normal serum osmolality and no significant reduction of urine volume during a carefully controlled fluid deprivation test. The primary polydipsia syndromes, by contrast, exhibit a low or low/normal serum osmolality and a sharp reduction in urine flow on fluid deprivation.

Table 3.

Primary polyuria	Primary polydipsia
Impaired ability to secrete ADH	Compulsive water drinking (psychogenic polydipsia)
Diabetes insipidus	
Target organ insensitivity to ADH	Hypothalamic disease
Nephrogenic diabetes insipidus	Hypokalaemia
	Hypercalcaemia
Osmotic diuresis	
Diabetes mellitus	
Hypercalciuria	
Solute administration	
Renal tubular defects	
Chronic pyelonephritis	
Chronic renal failure	
Hypokalaemia	
Hypercalcaemia	
Sickle cell disease	

78

Pituitary tumours

Pituitary tumours may be associated with acromegaly, gigantism, Cushing's disease and galactorrhoea, or they may be apparently non-secretory. The clinical importance of many pituitary tumours results from the pressure on normal pituitary tissue and adjacent structures, rather than their inherent secretory capacity. They may be chromophobic or chromophilic adenomas or craniopharyngiomas. Chromophobe and chromophil tumours are rare in childhood and may be associated with parathyroid and pancreatic tumours (see pages 212 and 218). Craniopharyngiomas are more common in childhood and adolescence (although they may not present until adult life) and may be detected radiologically by calcification in the tumour. The more recent term 'functionless pituitary tumour' is open to question, because many are associated with excessive prolactin secretion (even though galactorrhoea may not be present), and others secrete LH, FSH or α-subunits. **79** shows a pituitary tumour being dissected out at autopsy and **80** a tumour with a suprasellar extension. **81** shows a sagittal section of the pituitary with a microadenoma in the anterior lobe.

79

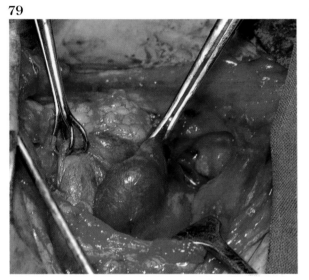

81

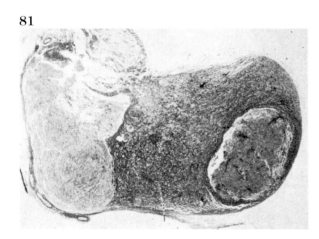

80

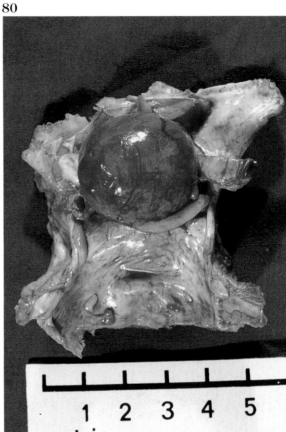

Pituitary tumours may be located within the pituitary fossa or extend laterally or above the sella turcica. Lateral radiographs of the skull may show expansion of the fossa, thinning of the walls, asymmetry or ballooning of the floor and/or erosion of the clinoid processes (**82**). Rarely, pituitary adenomas may contain calcified areas (**83**). The extent of a pituitary tumour can be demonstrated by CT scan or by magnetic resonance imaging. **84** shows a pituitary tumour with a suprasellar extension and thinning of the floor of the fossa on CT scan, and **85** a large tumour on the right displacing the pituitary stalk to the left. **86** and **87** show a craniopharyngioma with calcification on skull radiograph and CT scan. **88** demonstrates a pituitary tumour and **89** a hypothalamic tumour, both by magnetic resonance imaging. (**89** is reproduced by permission of the *Journal of the Royal Society of Medicine,* 1987; **80**: 707–708.)

82

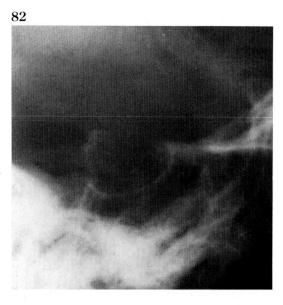

83

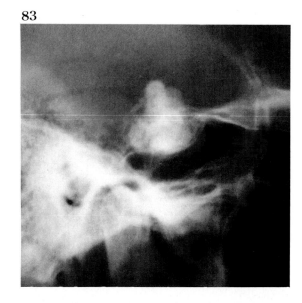

84

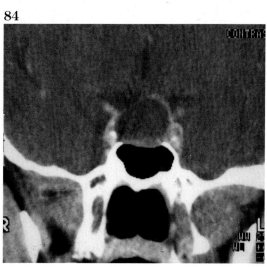

85

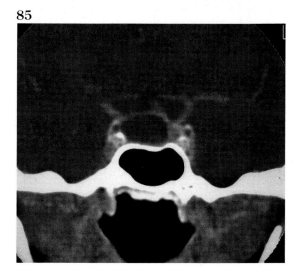

86

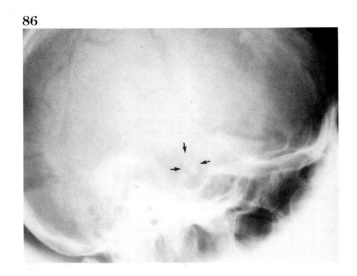

87

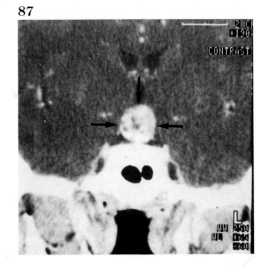

88

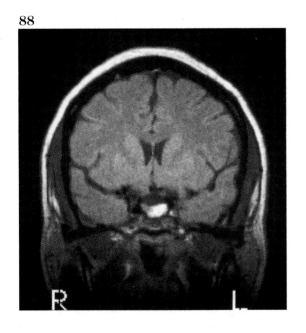

89

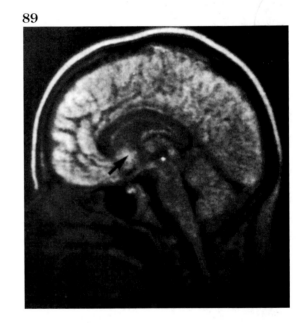

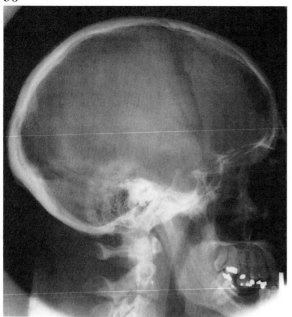

Compression of normal pituitary tissue may lead to impairment of endocrine function. Haemorrhage into a pituitary tumour may lead to acute pituitary insufficiency and this may be associated with sudden loss of vision and meningeal symptoms. Paradoxically an 'empty fossa' (the late consequence of infarction or a congenital deficiency in the diaphragma sellae) may be associated with surprisingly normal pituitary function (**90** shows an enlarged pituitary fossa on a skull radiograph, **91** a CT scan with only the centrally placed pituitary stalk visible and **92** a scan with contrast medium filling the empty fossa). Visual field defects are present in some patients. An upper quadrantic defect or hemianopia are most commonly seen. Asymmetrical expansion of the tumour occasionally leads to a unilateral field defect. Oculomotor palsies (e.g. IIIrd nerve palsy — **93** to **95**) are rare and papilloedema is very rare (**96**). Optic atrophy (**97**) may result from long-standing suprasellar extension with compression of optic pathways.

91

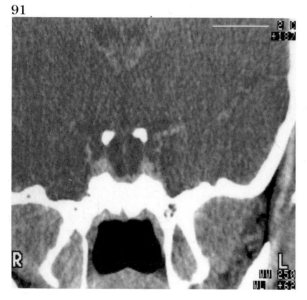

92

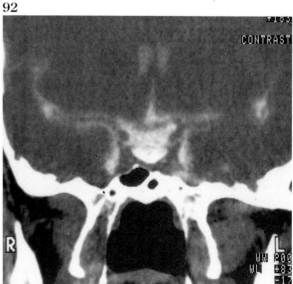

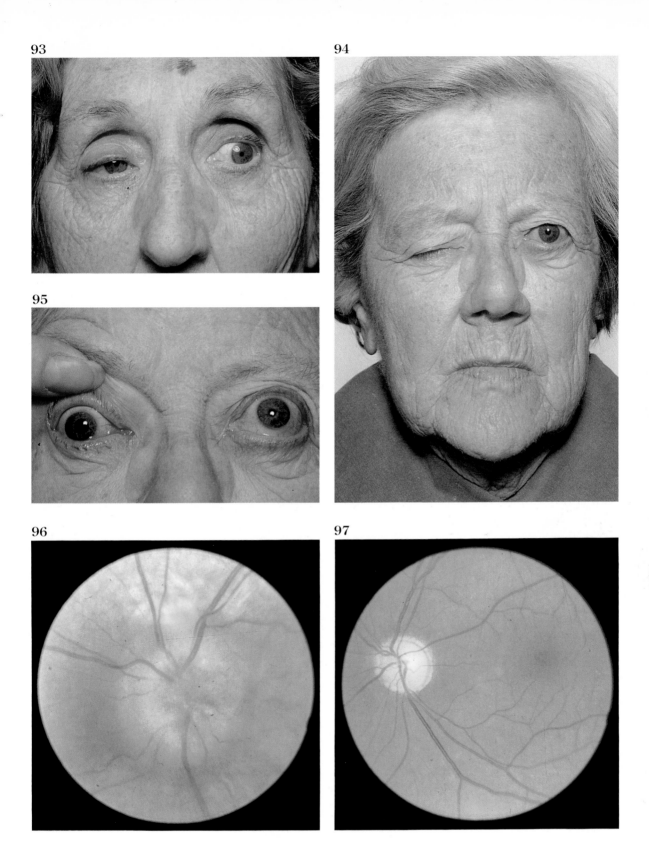

Miscellaneous hypothalamic disorders

A number of rare hypothalamic syndromes have been described. These include the following:

- **Hypothalamic obesity (98 to 100).**

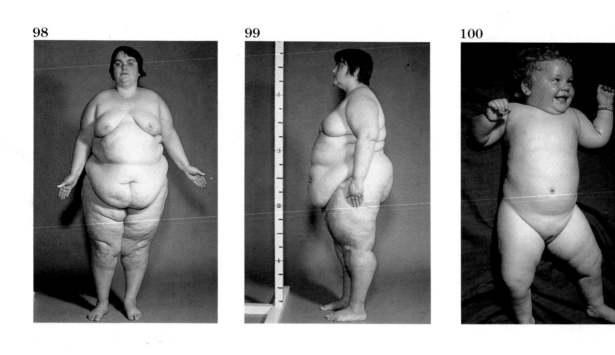

- **Lawrence–Moon–Biedl syndrome** (obesity 101, mental retardation, polydactyly 102 and 103, and hypogonadism 104).

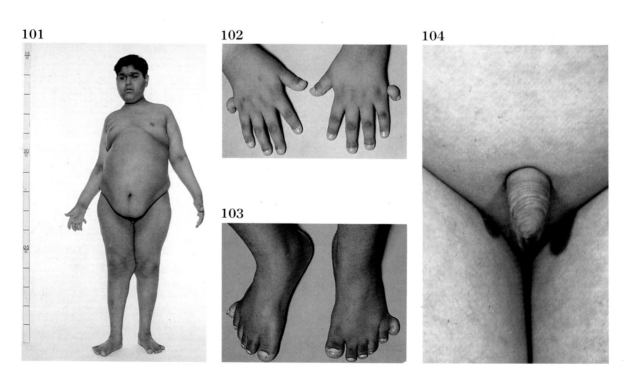

- **Histiocytosis X** (granulomatous deposits containing histiocytes **105**, in the hypothalamus, pituitary, orbit **106**, skull **107**, bones **108** and **109**, and lungs **110**).

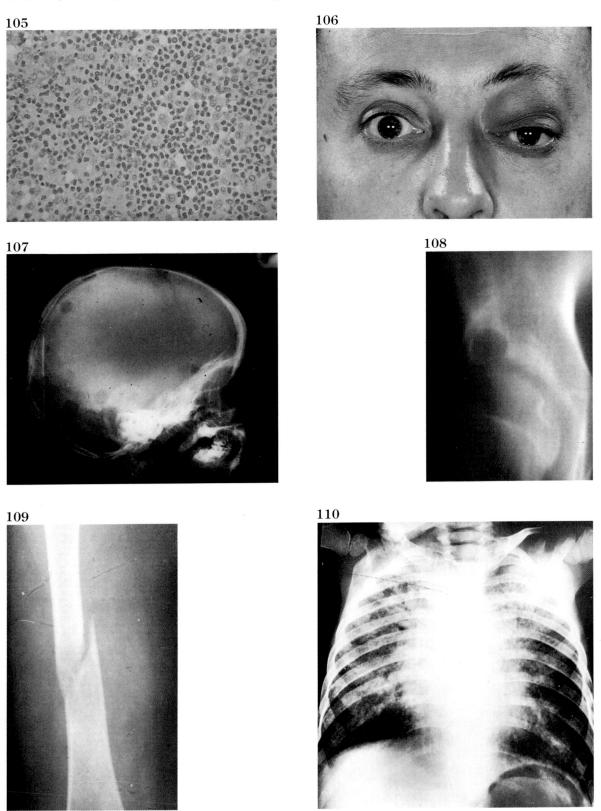

105

106

107

108

109

110

111

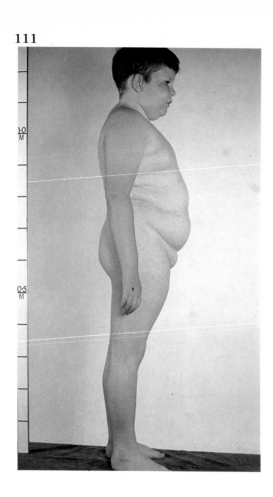

- **Prader–Willi syndrome** (gross obesity often complicated by diabetes **111**, small hands and small genitalia **112**; see also pages 47 and 211).

112

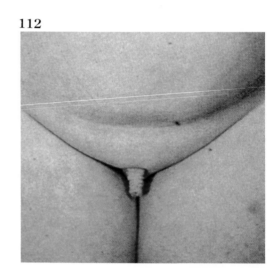

- **Polyostotic fibrous dysplasia** (**113** and **114**; see also pages 161 and 241) showing typical pigmentation.

113

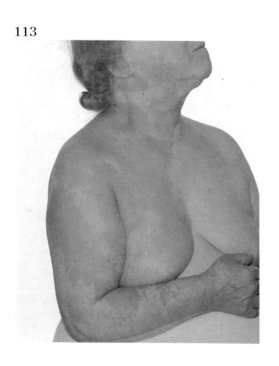

114

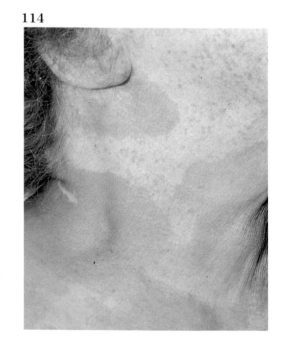

Chapter 2
Disorders of growth

Introduction

Normal growth results from an interplay of many intrinsic and extrinsic factors on the innate, genetically determined capacity for growth of the body cells. Growth and development proceed concomitantly in the normal child but these processes are to some extent independent and are under different hormonal and metabolic controls. Growth in height is the variable which is most easily observed, but alterations in skeletal proportions, maturation of the features, dental development and skeletal maturation must all be considered when assessing growth and development.

The final height attained by any individual depends not only on the rate of linear growth but also upon its duration and thus actual height at any age should always be assessed in the light of bone maturity or bone age.

Evaluation of growth

Height

Charts relating height to age indicate the rate of growth by comparison with a reference population. It must be remembered that genetic, racial and nutritional factors have a considerable influence on height and growth rate in the absence of any abnormality of growth. The most appropriate standards for height in the UK are the centile charts of Tanner and Whitehouse,* but other standards must be used for groups with a different racial background. The use of mid-parental height charts make allowance for genetic influences and permit correlation between a child's height and the mean height of both parents. Serial measurements of height may be compared with normal by the use of growth velocity charts. Abnormal height cannot be defined absolutely, but a child is usually considered short if his or her height is below the 3rd centile, or unduly tall if above the 97th centile — i.e. approximately two standard deviations below or above the mean.

Most people with **short stature** are not suffering from endocrine or other disease. The cause can usually be determined by the clinical features and a limited number of investigations. Particular attention should be paid to the family history of growth and development, the patient's birth weight and length, the pattern of growth in height and epiphyseal development, facial features, secondary sexual characteristics, dental

115

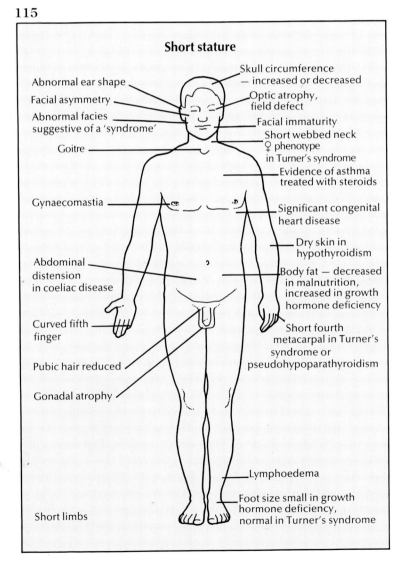

Short stature

Abnormal ear shape
Facial asymmetry
Abnormal facies suggestive of a 'syndrome'
Goitre
Gynaecomastia
Abdominal distension in coeliac disease
Curved fifth finger
Pubic hair reduced
Gonadal atrophy
Short limbs

Skull circumference — increased or decreased
Optic atrophy, field defect
Facial immaturity
Short webbed neck ♀ phenotype in Turner's syndrome
Evidence of asthma treated with steroids
Significant congenital heart disease
Dry skin in hypothyroidism
Body fat — decreased in malnutrition, increased in growth hormone deficiency
Short fourth metacarpal in Turner's syndrome or pseudohypoparathyroidism
Lymphoedema
Foot size small in growth hormone deficiency, normal in Turner's syndrome

---

* A variety of growth charts is available from Castlemead Publications, Castlemead, Gascoyne Way, Hertford SG14 1LH, UK.

41

development, body weight, appetite and nutrition, infections and previous diseases, and intelligence. The clinical features which may be associated with short stature are shown in **115**. Investigations may include urinalysis, blood count and erythrocyte sedimentation rate, chromosomal analysis (karyotype), radiographs of chest and skull, left hand and wrist (bone age), left knee (state of epiphyseal fusion), and other more specialised endocrine tests as indicated.

Tall stature is a much less common medical problem than short stature. Most tall children and adults fall into the group with familial tall stature, particularly if both parents are tall. They are well, and their height falls within the normal range when allowance is made for mid-parental height and their growth runs above and parallel to the 97th centile. Their final height may be predicted from the tables of Bayer and Bayley[†] on the basis of their skeletal maturation.

Skeletal proportions

Assessment of skeletal proportions is an essential part of the evaluation of growth disorders. The most straightforward clinical observation is the measurement of lower and upper segments. The lower segment,

---

[†] Bayer LM, Bayley N. *Growth Diagnosis*. Chicago: University of Chicago Press, USA, 1959.

measured in the standing position, is the distance from the top of the symphysis pubis to the floor, and the length of the upper segment is obtained by subtraction of the lower segment from the total height. The limbs are relatively short in early life, and thus the lower segment is relatively short, but by 10 or 11 years of age the growth of the limbs causes the ratio of the upper and lower segments to reach unity and this ratio remains static into adult life.

Proportionate dwarfism generally results from chromosomal, endocrine, metabolic, nutritional or psychosocial abnormalities. There may, however, be differences within this group. Hypothyroid dwarfs retain infantile proportions and thus have a high upper to lower segment ratio. **116** shows a hypothyroid boy with an age-matched control. The upper to lower segment ratio is normal in other forms of proportionate dwarfism. Excessive linear growth may result from endocrine, chromosomal or metabolic abnormalities and is not generally associated with a major degree of skeletal disproportion. Measurement of the span may be helpful because it largely reflects the length of the arms and is more than 5 cm greater than the height in patients with eunuchoid proportions (e.g. Klinefelter's syndrome) and in Marfan's syndrome.

Disproportionate dwarfism may result from a variety of inherited skeletal dysplasias or as a result of acquired disease of the skeleton. The skeletal dysplasias are normally classified as 'short limb' or 'short trunk' according to the nature of the skeletal disproportion.

116

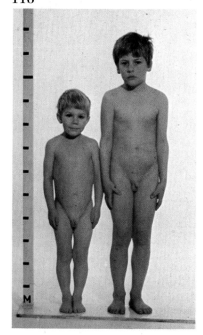

117

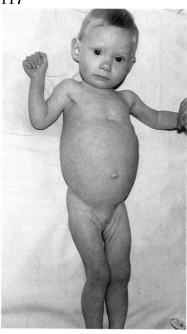

118

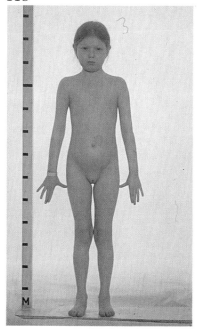

Weight

The relation of weight to age in the two sexes can be obtained from Tanner and Whitehouse charts. If growth is impaired by malnutrition, weight is likely to be reduced to a greater extent than height. **117** and **118** show malnourished short children with intestinal malabsorption.

Maturation of features

Facial appearance is an important guide to skeletal maturity. Growth of the bridge of the nose is impaired during infancy and thus accounts for the characteristically immature face of the cretin (**119**).

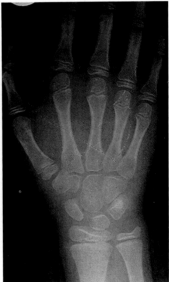

Bone maturation

Bone age is best determined radiologically. Radiographs of the hand and wrist can be compared with plates depicting the degree of skeletal development of healthy children at different ages. For Western communities the reader is referred to the *Radiographic Atlas of Skeletal Development of the Hand and Wrist* by Greulich WW and Pyle SI (1959). A skeletal age more than two standard deviations below the mean makes it highly probable that the child's bone maturation is abnormally retarded. **120** shows a radiograph of the left hand and wrist from a normal 11-year-old girl (left) and a radiograph from a growth hormone deficient child of the same age and sex.

120

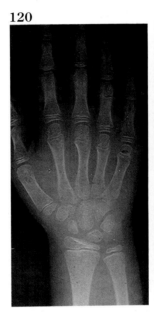

Dental development

The basic growth may be assessed by inspection or by dental radiographs. Both primary and secondary dentition are affected by similar factors to those affecting bone maturation.

Short stature

Patients with normal proportions

Those with normal proportions make up the majority of children with short stature.

Congenital causes

Familial shortness may occur alone or in combination with delayed development, which is often also familial. This is by far the commonest cause of short stature. Diagnosis is usually established from the family history. Charts correlating the child's height and mid-parental height may be helpful. Gross shortness is seen in the rare syndrome of primordial dwarfism. **121** and **122** show an affected child and an age- and sex-matched control.

Children with **low birth weight dwarfism** constitute a heterogeneous group, and the condition may be associated with a wide variety of major and minor congenital anomalies including an odd facies, ptosis, an incurved little finger or a high-arched palate. An abnormal pregnancy producing an unhealthy placenta is a further cause of low birth weight dwarfism and may lead to prolonged or even permanent shortness of stature. **123** shows monozygotic twins of dissimilar birth weight at 7½ years of age. Other causes include intrauterine infections (e.g. rubella or toxoplasmosis) or chromosomal anomalies. **124** shows a child with intrauterine growth retardation caused by congenital virus infection (rubella) which has also led to hepato-splenomegaly, shown by the skin markings, and thrombocytopenia. Autosomal chromosomal anomalies such as Trisomy 9 (**125**) or some other disorders, not all of which are readily identifiable, may also cause intrauterine growth retardation.

121

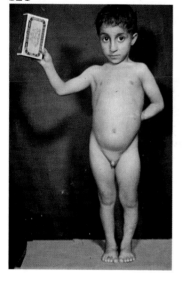

122

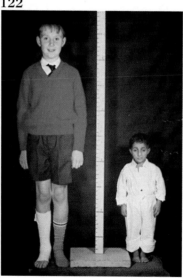

123

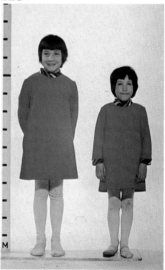

124

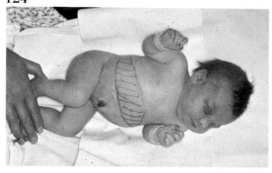

125

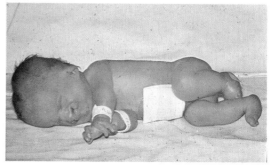

Many other syndromes may be associated with shortness of stature. These are well illustrated by Smith (1970).* They should be considered if the child has an odd facies, mental retardation or a low birth weight. Russell–Silver syndrome shows a normal skull circumference for age and some asymmetry of body growth (**126**). The facial asymmetry and shortness in this condition are illustrated in figures **127** to **129** (with an age- and sex-matched control in **129**), and abnormalities of the hand and foot in **130** and **131**. Associated precocious puberty may cause acceleration of growth.

* Smith DW. *Recognisable Patterns of Human Malformation.* Philadelphia and London: W. B. Saunders, 1970.

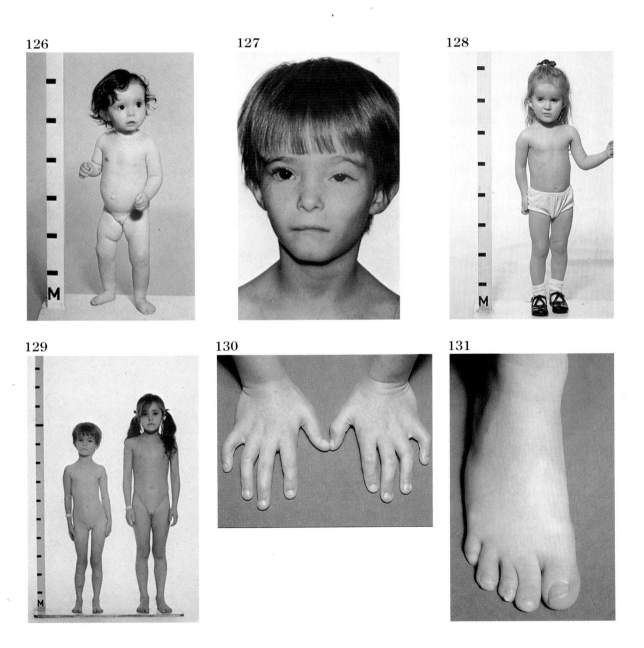

126

127

128

129

130

131

Children with **Hallerman–Streiff syndrome** are short, suffer from brachycephaly with frontal and parietal bossing, micrognathia, microphthalmia and a thin, pointed nose 132 to 134.

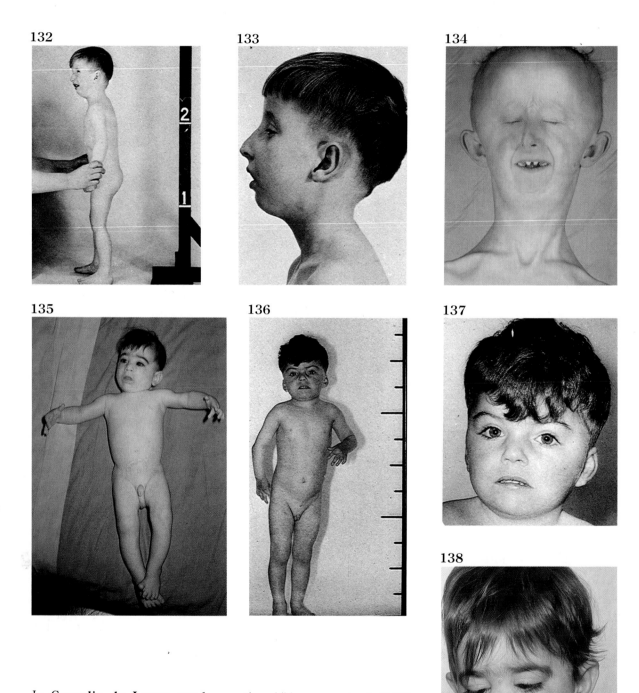

132

133

134

135

136

137

138

In **Cornelia de Lange syndrome** the children are short (135), mentally retarded with brachycephaly, have bushy eyebrows, long curly eyelashes, a small nose with anteverted nostrils, and micrognathia (136 to 138).

139

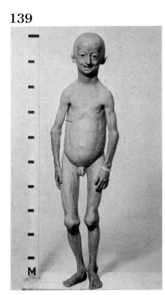

140

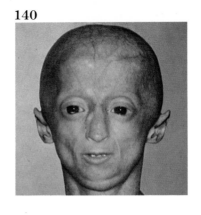

141

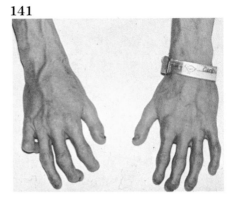

142

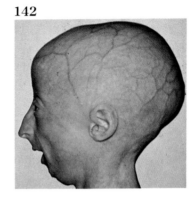

139 to **142** show a child with **progeria** illustrating the alopecia, thin skin, atrophy of the subcutaneous fat, skeletal hypoplasia causing shortness, peri-articular fibrosis and arthritis with stiff, partially flexed, swollen joints.

143

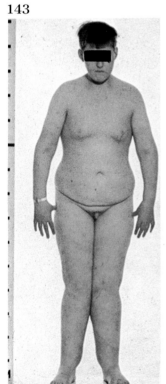

In **Prader–Willi syndrome** shortness is associated with gross obesity, mental retardation, small hands and feet, underdeveloped genitalia and later carbohydrate intolerance and diabetes mellitus (**143** to **145**).

144

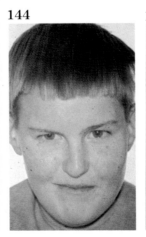

145

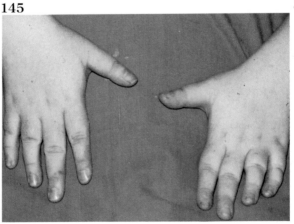

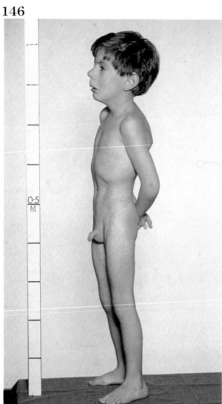

146

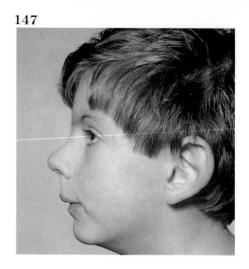

147

Seckel's syndrome consists of facial hypoplasia, a prominent nose, microcephaly, multiple minor joint abnormalities and mental retardation associated with shortness of normal proportions (**146** and **147**).

Patients with **Ollier's disease** have an abnormal pattern of growth of unossified cartilage affecting the long bones with multiple exostoses (**148**).

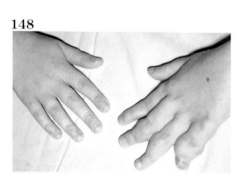

148

Aarskog's syndrome comprises hypertelorism, small hands and feet, interdigital webbing and a scrotal shawl above the penis. The children are short and inheritance is X-linked (**149** and **150**).

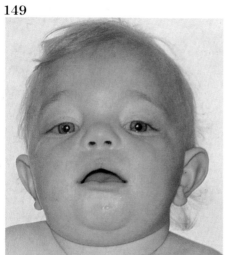

149

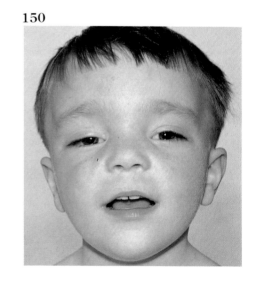

150

In **William's syndrome** there are full lips, a small nose with anteverted nostrils, dysplasia of the iris, hypoplasia of the nails, hypercalcaemia in infancy, supravalvular aortic stenosis and shortness **151** and **152**. The pattern of inheritance is not known.

151

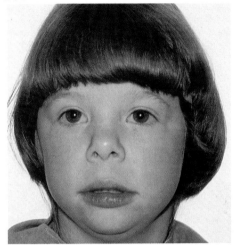

152

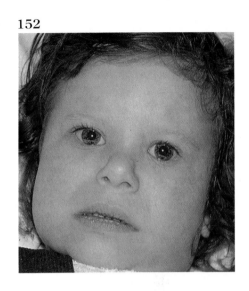

Dwarfism is also associated with the **mucopolysaccharidoses** — a large group of biochemical storage disorders caused by lysosomal enzyme defects. The three most commonly seen (although all are rare) are **Morquio's syndrome**, **Hurler's syndrome** and **Hunter's syndrome**. Morquio's syndrome is an autosomal recessive condition marked by severe growth retardation associated with joint deformities (particularly genu valgum) and normal intelligence (**153**). **154** shows the bone changes associated with mucopolysaccharidosis. Odontoid hypoplasia may lead to atlanto-axial subluxation with spinal cord compression. Dwarfism is also severe in Hurler's syndrome, which is also an autosomal recessive, and is associated with hepatosplenomegaly, abdominal protuberance, umbilical hernia, joint contractures and mental retardation. Impairment of growth tends to be less severe in Hunter's syndrome (an X-linked recessive), and is associated with hepatosplenomegaly, umbilical hernia and normal intelligence.

153

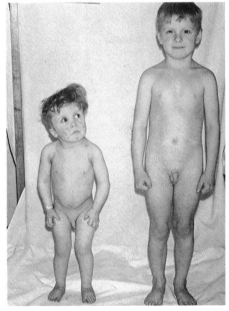

154

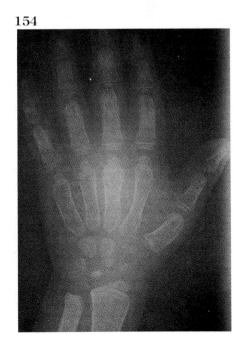

Nutritional disorders

The commonest cause of pathological shortness of stature worldwide is malnutrition, and social, agricultural, economic and infective factors may all contribute to the clinical picture. Kwashiorkor is caused by gross protein deficiency, generally associated with a high carbohydrate intake. It is characterised by generalised oedema, areas of skin pigmentation alternating with scaling areas of decreased pigmentation, and loss of pigment from the hair (**155** to **157**). Marasmus results from severe calorie malnutrition leading to wasting and shortness of stature (**158**). **159** shows a marasmic child aged 3½ years on the left compared with a normal child aged 10 months.

Gross malnutrition is uncommon in developed countries but may result from malabsorption, psychological disorders, chronic infections or severe socio-economic problems. Malabsorption syndromes may be overlooked because anaemia, a large abdomen and a tendency to diarrhoea may not be obvious (**160**). Subcutaneous fat may be retained although muscle wasting is usually present.

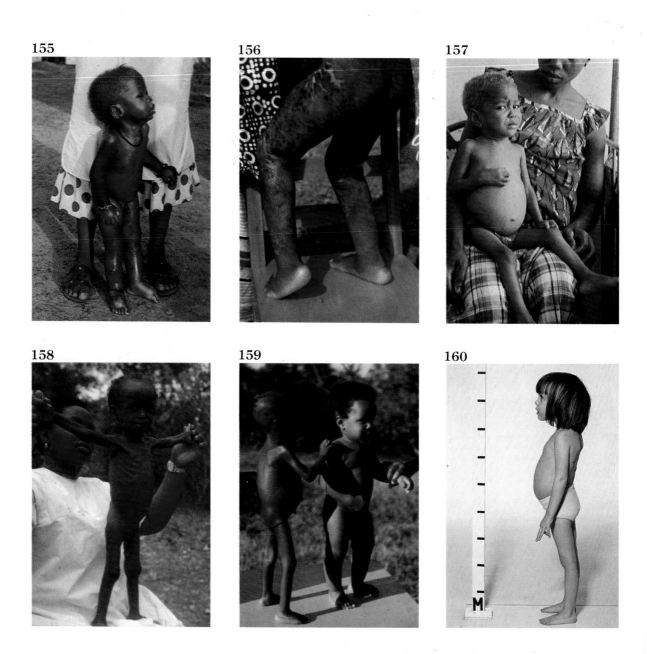

Systemic disease

Any disease affecting a major organ or system may lead to impaired growth and development. Chronic renal disease (**161**), cyanotic congenital heart disease, prolonged anaemia or mental retardation may all be associated with shortness.

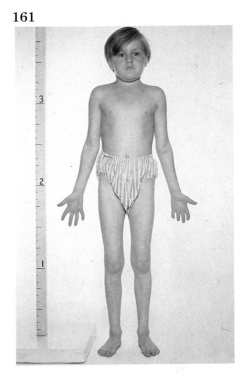

Endocrine disorders

Growth hormone deficiency (see also Chapter 1). Congenital or acquired deficiency of growth hormone secretion or action in childhood will lead to shortness of stature. The children are usually plump with immature facies and genitalia and delicate extremities (**162** and **163**).

162

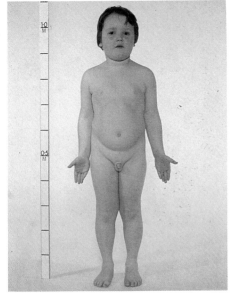

163

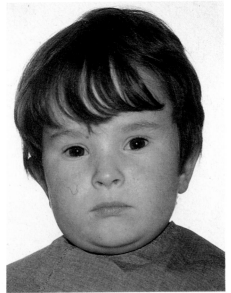

164 shows two siblings, a 15-year-old boy and a 13-year-old girl, with familial isolated growth hormone deficiency, and **165** shows a 9-year-old pituitary dwarf compared with an age- and sex-matched control. A micropenis (**166** and **167**) is present in one-third of boys with isolated growth hormone deficiency.

164

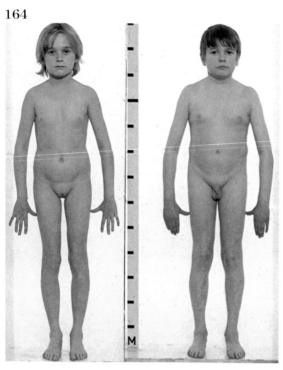

165

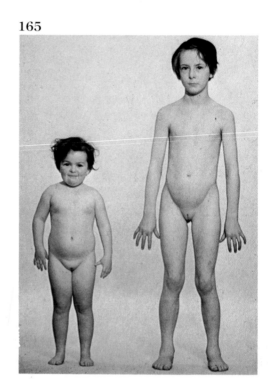

166

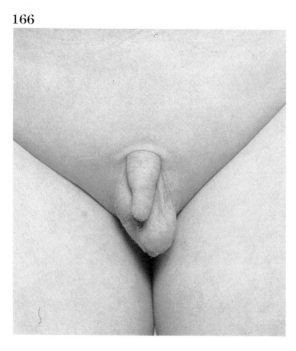

167

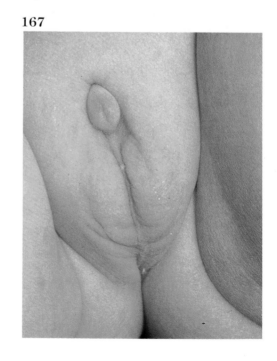

168

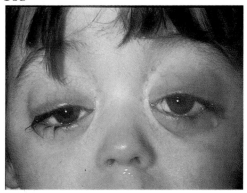

169

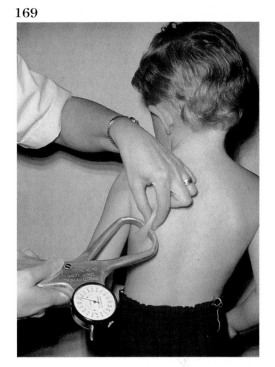

Organic causes of growth hormone deficiency include histiocytosis X, shown here affecting the orbit (**168**).

The increased subcutaneous fat can be demonstrated by measuring the subscapular skinfold thickness (**169**). This decreases on treatment with growth hormone.

Hypothyroidism (see also Chapter 3). Thyroid failure should always be suspected in short children and the earlier its onset the more severe the delay in growth and skeletal maturation. Body proportions remain infantile and bone age is retarded more than height.

170 shows a short hypothyroid child, and **171** shows comparison with an age- and sex-matched control. Bone age lags behind chronological age. **172** shows the wrist of a hypothyroid child aged 3 years with a bone age of 6 months.

170

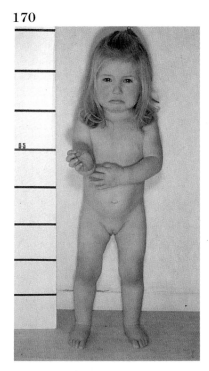

171

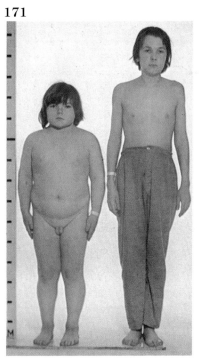

172

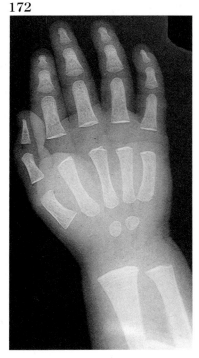

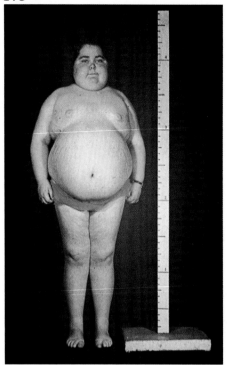 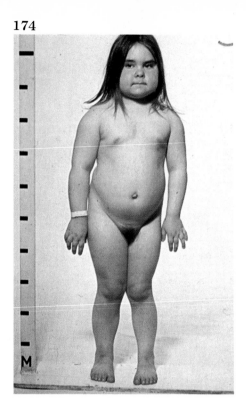

Cushing's syndrome (see also Chapter 4). Cushing's syndrome is always associated with growth retardation in childhood (**173** shows severe Cushing's syndrome caused by steroid therapy) and normal growth excludes this diagnosis. **174** shows a short child with Cushing's syndrome caused by an adrenal adenoma.

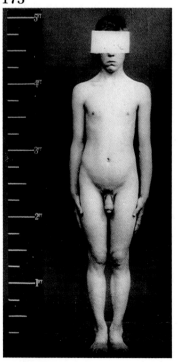

Congenital adrenal hyperplasia (see also Chapter 4). Excessive androgen production causes increased linear growth in early life, but this is associated with precocious puberty and early skeletal maturation leading to premature epiphyseal fusion, and thus final height is reduced. **175** shows a tall boy (aged 8 years) with precocious sexual development and hypertension caused by 11 ß-hydroxylase deficiency.

Sexual precocity. True precocious puberty or sexual precocity resulting from androgen- or estrogen-secreting tumours is associated with excessive skeletal growth and enhanced rate of maturation and thus final height is reduced.

Emotional deprivation. This is an important cause of failure to thrive and shortness of stature. The facial appearance, behaviour and intellect are immature and the abdomen may be protuberant (**176**). Bone age is retarded in proportion to the reduced height. Responses of growth hormone and ACTH to appropriate stimuli are deficient but return to normal in a secure environment. **177** shows an emotionally deprived child with an age- and sex-matched control.

176

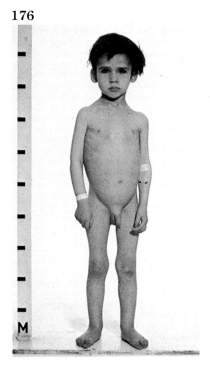

177

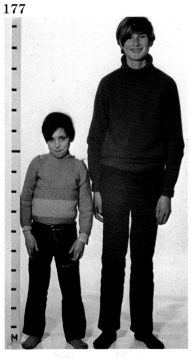

178

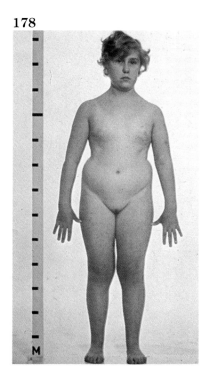

179

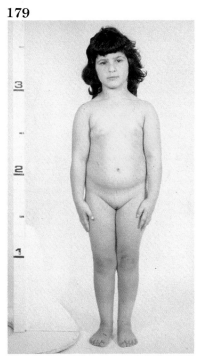

180

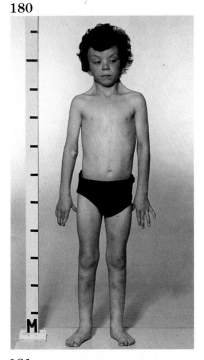

181

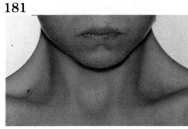

Sex chromosome anomalies (see also Chapter 5). Turner's syndrome (karyotype 45,XO) or one of its many chromosomal variants is always associated with short stature and delayed development. **178** shows a 16-year-old girl with short stature, primary amenorrhoea and lack of secondary sexual characteristics caused by XO/XY Turner's mosaicism. The characteristic somatic and radiological changes are easily recognised. **179** illustrates short stature associated with a ring chromosome 15, and **180** and **181** short stature and webbing of the neck in Noonan's syndrome (see also page 144).

Patients with abnormal proportions

Shortness of stature with abnormal proportions is uncommon but may be associated with gross stunting. Most cases result from skeletal dysplasias which are of genetic origin. It is common to separate these disorders into 'short limb' and 'short trunk' varieties. It should be remembered that the skeletal dysplasias form a very large and heterogeneous group of disorders which may be associated with a wide range of clinical features, and many of them have been identified by a variety of names in the past. More complete descriptions of these and the other syndromes in this group can be found in 'The chondrodysplasias' by

Rimoin DL and Lachman RS, in *Principles and Practice of Medical Genetics,* Emery AEH and Rimoin DL (eds). Edinburgh and London: Churchill Livingstone, 1983.

Short limb dwarfism

The major varieties of short limb dwarfism are shown in Table 4. Most of the skeletal dysplasias are extremely rare. The most common is achondroplasia which occurs with a frequency of 1 in 40,000 births in western societies.

Table 4. Varieties of short limb dwarfism.

Syndrome	Inheritance	Manifestations
Achondroplasia (**182** to **184**)	Autosomal dominant	Large head and short limbs; distinct milder types occur

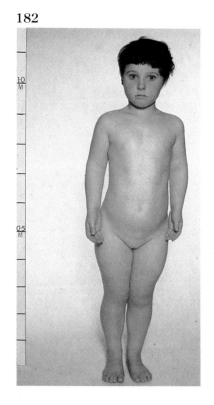

182

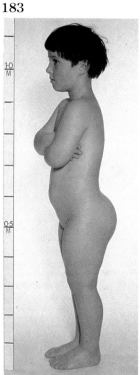

183

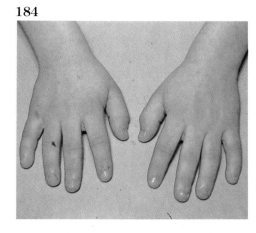

184

Table 4 (continued).

Syndrome	Inheritance	Manifestations
Hypochondroplasia (**185**)	Autosomal dominant	Mild dwarfism; mental retardation in 10%
Diastrophic dwarfism (**186** and **187**)	Recessive	Limitation of joints; club foot; scoliosis
Thanatophoric dwarfism (**188** to **190**)	? Recessive	Very short limbs and small chest; all die as neonates

185

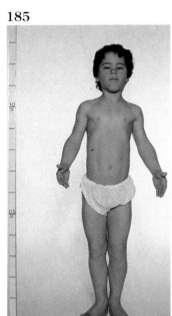

186

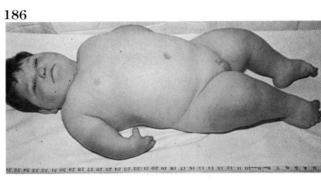

187

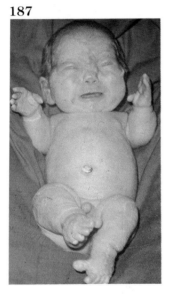

188

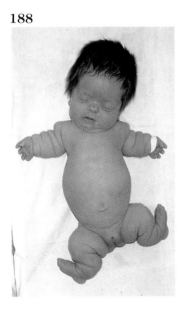

189

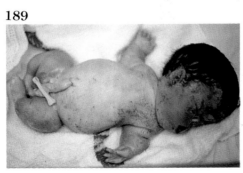

190

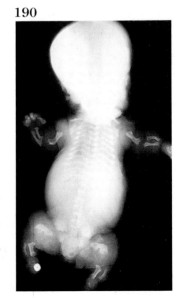

Table 4 (continued).

Syndrome	Inheritance	Manifestations
Metatrophic dwarfism (**191**)	Uncertain	Short limbs, small epiphyses, severe kyphoscoliosis
Achondrogenesis (2 variants)	Recessive	Grossly deficient calcification; all die as neonates
Pseudoachondroplasia	Dominant or (rarely) recessive	Joint deformities, laxity of ligaments and contractures
Metaphyseal chondrodysplasia	a) Recessive	McKusick type — fine, sparse hair; scalloped metaphyses
	b) Dominant	Schmid type — mild dwarfism with bowing of limbs
	c) Dominant	Jansen type — short limbs, large joints
Chondrodysplasia punctata (**192** and **193**)	a) Dominant b) Recessive c) X-linked dominant	Conradi–Hünerman type Rhizomelic type
Chondroectodermal dysplasia (**194** and **195**)	Recessive	Ellis–van Creveld syndrome — congenital heart lesions, hypoplastic nails and teeth

191

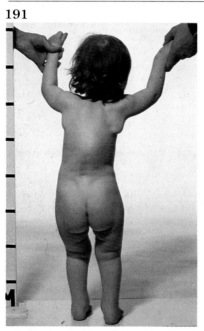

192

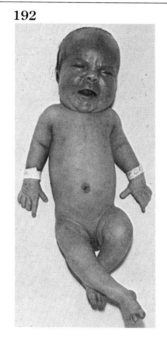

193

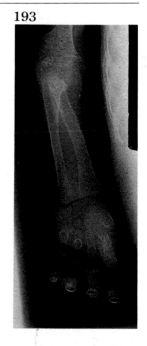

194

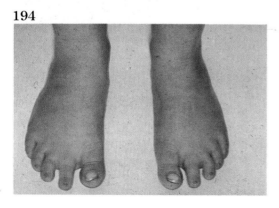

195

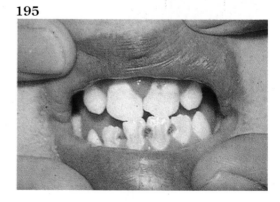

Table 4 (continued).

Syndrome	Inheritance	Manifestations
Grebe chondrodysplasia	Recessive	Severe distal limb deficit
Acromesomelic dysplasia	Recessive	Severe dwarfism
Multiple epiphyseal dysplasia (**196** to **203**)	Dominant (commonly) or recessive	Moderate stunting of growth (Fairbank syndrome)
Pycnodysostosis	Recessive	Hyperostosis, mild dwarfism and delayed dentition
Campomelic dysplasia (3 variants)	Recessive or unknown	Prenatal bowing of limbs; tracheomalacia

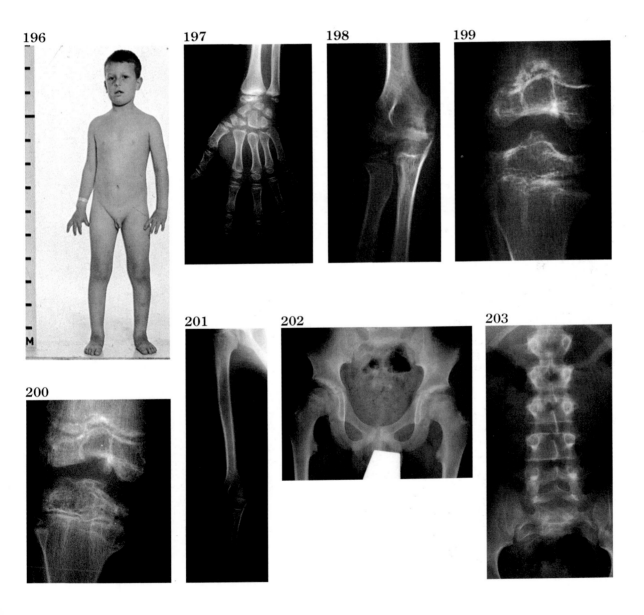

196

197

198

199

201

202

203

200

Table 4 (continued).

Syndrome	Inheritance	Manifestations
Hypophosphataemic rickets	X-linked dominant	Bowing of legs, vitamin D resistance
Hypophosphatasia	Recessive Dominant or recessive	Congenital lethal variety Hypophosphatasia tarda
Osteogenesis imperfecta (**204** to **207**)	Autosomal dominant Types I and IV Autosomal recessive Types II and III	Bowing of legs, blue sclerae, frequent fractures, hypoplastic teeth. Variable features according to different genetic syndromes

204

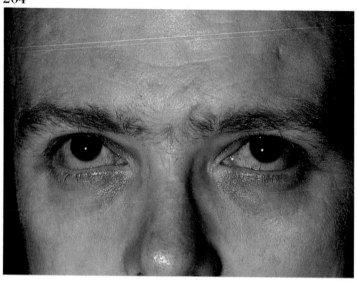

205

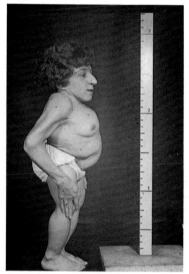

206

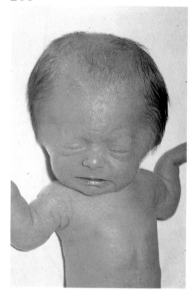

207

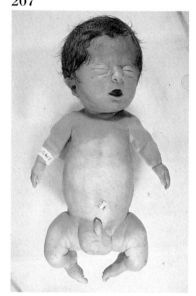

Short trunk dwarfism

The short trunk varieties of dwarfism are even more rare than the short limb varieties and the principal features are shown in Table 5.

Table 5. Varieties of short trunk dwarfism.

Syndrome	Inheritance	Manifestations
Spondyloepiphyseal dysplasia tarda	X-linked recessive, autosomal dominant or recessive	Late and relatively mild growth failure
Spondyloepiphyseal dysplasia congenita	Autosomal dominant	Very short trunk, flat face, myopia, retinal detachment
Spondylococcal dysostosis	Autosomal recessive or dominant	Short trunk, recessive forms more severe, chest infections
Dyggve–Melchior–Clausen dysplasia	Autosomal recessive	Early onset, abnormalities of joints and contractures, mental retardation
Kniest dysplasia	Autosomal dominant	Vertebral deformities, abnormal facies, myopia, hearing loss
Trichorhinophalangeal syndrome (**208**)	Autosomal dominant	Osteochondrodysplasia, bulbous nose, sparse hair, cone-shaped phalangeal epiphyses

208

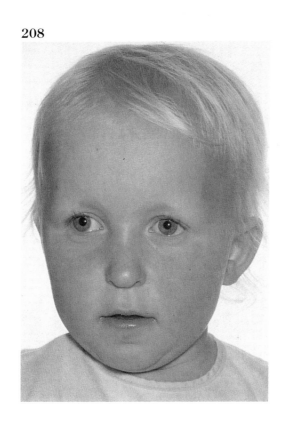

Tall stature

Tall stature is a much less common problem than short stature. Most cases result from familial tallness of stature. **209** shows a man referred with possible acromegaly, but when seen with his mother and sister (**210**) it is clear that he has familial tallness of stature. Overnutrition before puberty tends to increase a child's height as well as weight, but as bone age and puberty are also advanced the adult height is not increased. Advanced development is the opposite of physiologically delayed puberty; it is often familial with rapid growth and advanced bone age throughout childhood but final height is normal.

209

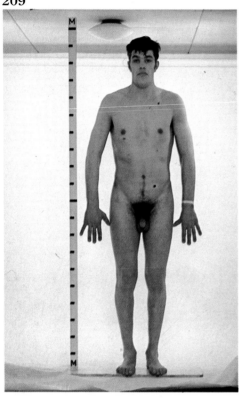

210

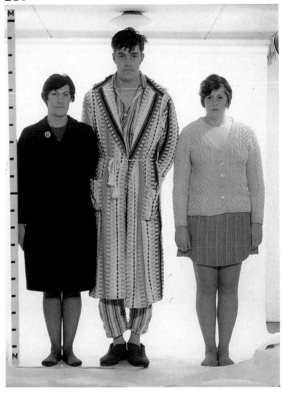

Endocrine disorders

Growth hormone excess

Growth hormone excess before puberty is very uncommon and some acromegalic features invariably accompany those of gigantism. **211** shows a 4½-year-old girl with gigantism and large broad hands and **212** her appearance at 15 years after successful treatment. **213** shows an 11-year-old boy with gigantism with an age-matched control, and **214** and **215** his large hands and feet compared with a control.

Sexual precocity

Sexual precocity from any cause is initially accompanied by an increase in linear growth, although final height is reduced as a result of premature fusion of the epiphyses.

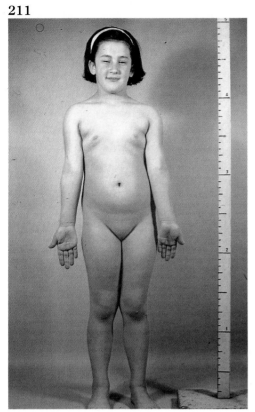

212

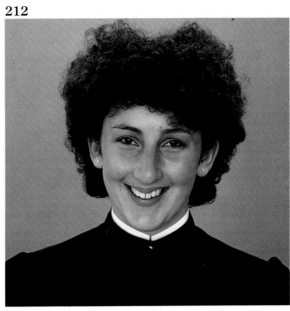

213

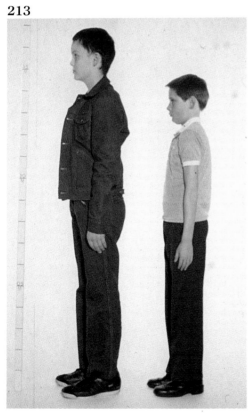

214

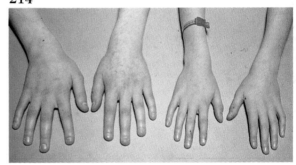

215

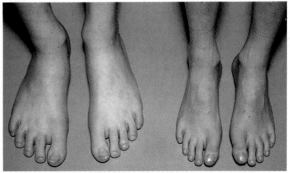

216

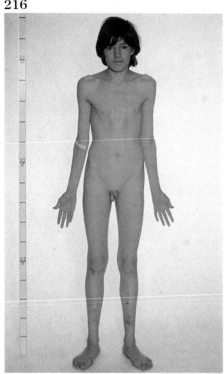

Eunuchoidism

Hypogonadism from any cause can produce an increase in growth resulting from delayed fusion of the epiphyses as long as growth hormone secretion is maintained. This can be seen in primary gonadal failure or in isolated gonadotrophin deficiency as in Kallmann's syndrome (**216**).

Hyperthyroidism

Hyperthyroidism in children produces an acceleration of growth rate with advanced bone age. Premature fusion of skull sutures can cause raised intracranial pressure.

Chromosomal disorders

Patients with Klinefelter's syndrome, 47,XXY (**217**), and those with the 47,XYY syndrome (**218**) are usually tall, although in the former this is largely the result of androgen deficiency.

217

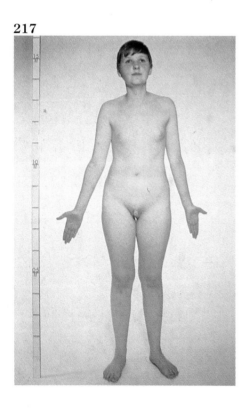

218

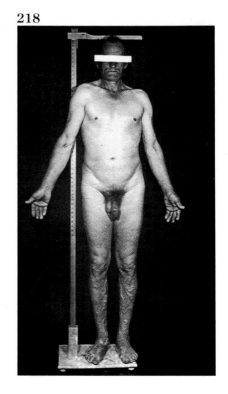

Miscellaneous disorders

A variety of disorders causing tall stature may be recognised, although most are rare. Children with **generalised lipodystrophy** may be tall. Patients with **Marfan's syndrome** are tall (**219**) and may be recognised by their numerous skeletal and somatic abnormalities. These include a high-arched palate, dislocated lenses, long fingers and toes (arachnodactyly), kyphoscoliosis and pectus excavatum (**220** to **223**).

219

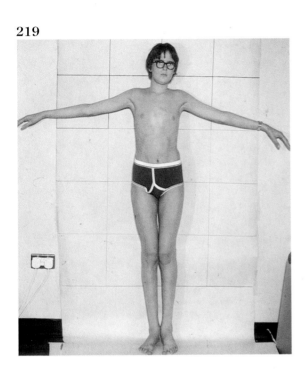

220

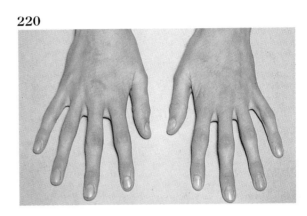

221

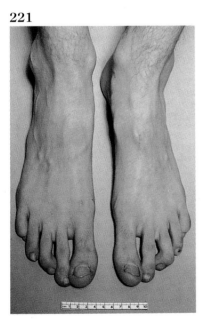

222

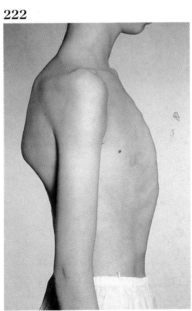

223

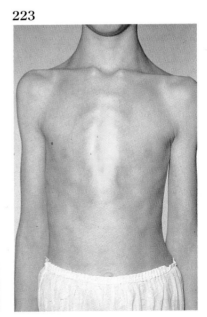

Soto's syndrome of cerebral gigantism (**224** and **225**) is associated with clumsiness, mental retardation (**226**), macrocrania, prognathism, dolichocephaly, high-arched palate, frontal bossing, hypertelorism, an anti-mongoloid obliquity of the palpebral fissures and hypogonadism (**227** and **228**).

The **exomphalos – macroglossia – gigantism syndrome** is a very rare familial syndrome and is associated with hypoglycaemia and intra-abdominal malignancy.

224

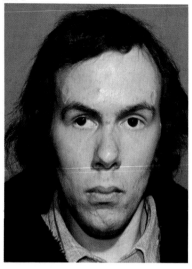

225

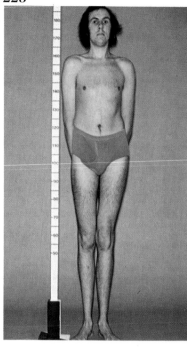

226

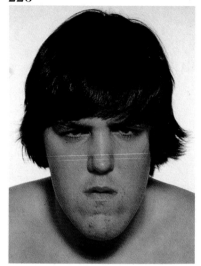

227

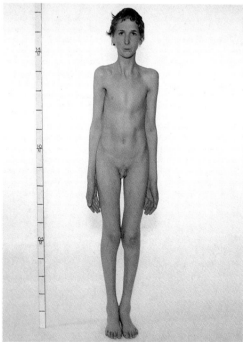

228

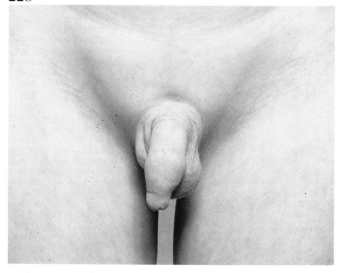

Chapter 3
Thyroid

Introduction

The thyroid gland secretes three hormones, thyroxine (T_4), triiodothyronine (T_3) and calcitonin. T_4 and T_3 are secreted by the follicular cells under the control of thyroid stimulating hormone which, after binding to a membrane receptor, activates adenylate cyclase. Calcitonin secretion is stimulated by elevation of the serum calcium, but its role in normal physiology remains uncertain.

Clinical features of thyroid disease

The three common presentations of thyroid disease are:

1.   Hyperthyroidism (**229**)

2.   Hypothyroidism (**230**)

3.   Goitre (**231**) which may be non-toxic or associated with hyperthyroidism or hypothyroidism.

229

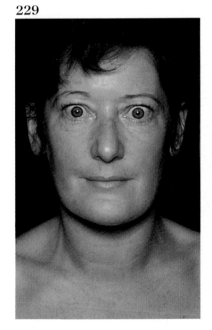

230

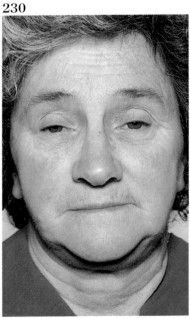

231

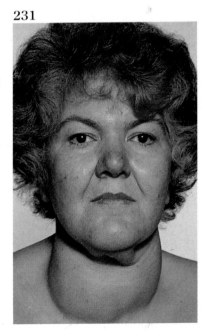

232

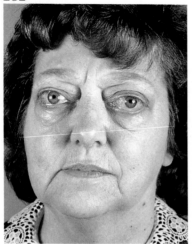

Hyperthyroidism

Hyperthyroidism is the clinical condition that results from increased circulating levels of free thyroid hormones. The causes of hyperthyroidism, listed in their approximate order of frequency in the UK include:

- Graves' disease (**232**)
- Toxic multinodular goitre (**233**)
- Toxic adenoma (**234**)
- Post-partum thyroiditis
- Jod–Basedow phenomenon
- De Quervain's thyroiditis
- Thyrotroph adenoma

- Excess thyroid hormone ingestion (iatrogenic, voluntary self-administration or from contaminated meat products)
- Molar hyperthyroidism
- Thyroid carcinoma
- Struma ovarii

Graves' disease

This is the commonest cause of hyperthyroidism. The major clinical features are shown in **235** and include:

- Hyperthyroidism
- Goitre
- Eye signs

- Localised myxoedema
- Thyroid acropachy
- Other associated features

233

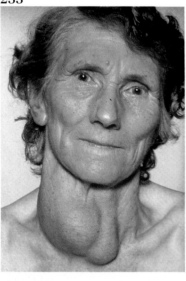

235

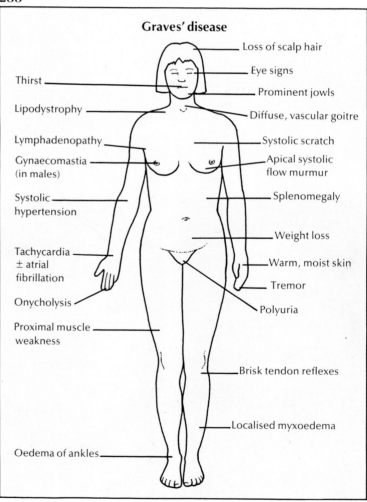

Graves' disease

Loss of scalp hair
Eye signs
Prominent jowls
Diffuse, vascular goitre
Systolic scratch
Apical systolic flow murmur
Splenomegaly
Weight loss
Warm, moist skin
Tremor
Polyuria
Brisk tendon reflexes
Localised myxoedema

Thirst
Lipodystrophy
Lymphadenopathy
Gynaecomastia (in males)
Systolic hypertension
Tachycardia ± atrial fibrillation
Onycholysis
Proximal muscle weakness
Oedema of ankles

234

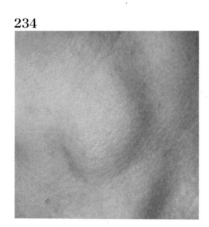

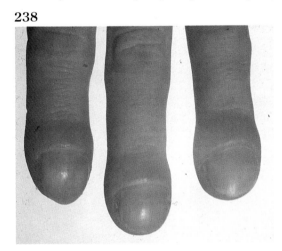

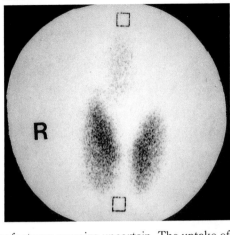

The goitre and hyperthyroidism of Graves' disease result from antibodies interacting with the thyrotrophin (TSH) receptor (TRAb) (**236**) but the pathogenesis of the other features remains uncertain. The uptake of radioiodine is characteristically diffuse (**237**).

Signs and symptoms of hyperthyroidism

The increased metabolic rate resulting from hyperthyroidism accounts for many of the clinical features of the condition. The palms are warm and moist, and the nails may exhibit acropachy. Thyroid acropachy resembles clubbing of the fingers and toes (**238**) but the oedema of the nail folds seen in the latter is inconspicuous (**239**) and the thumb and index fingers are most severely affected (**240, 241**).

238

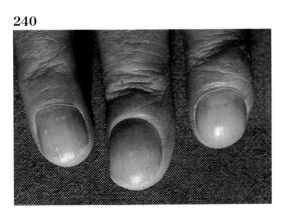

239

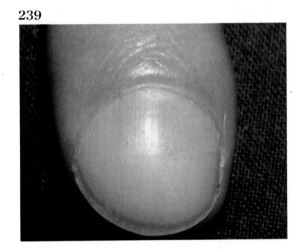

240

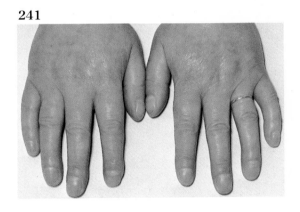

241

242 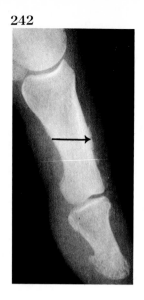 **243** 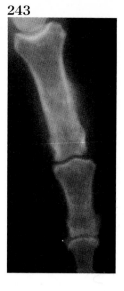 **244**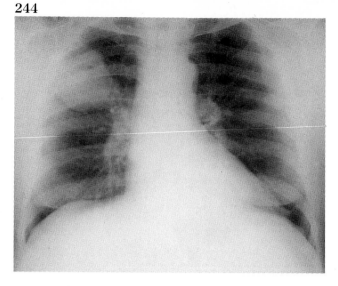

Radiographs of the hands and wrists may show patchy subperiosteal **new bone formation** resembling bubbles (**242** and **243**); this differs from the linear new bone formation seen in hypertrophic osteoarthropathy where a lung tumour is often visible on the chest radiograph (**244**).

245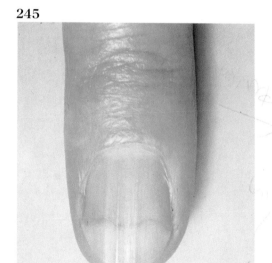

In **onycholysis** there is recession of the nails from the nail beds and the patient has difficulty in keeping the nails clean (**245** and **246**). A similar appearance is seen in some patients with psoriasis (**247**).

246 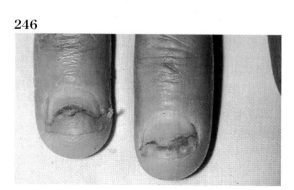 **247**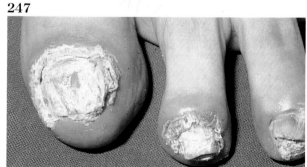

A fine **finger tremor** can be seen but is best appreciated by asking the patient to spread the fingers and rest them on the examiner's fingers (**248**). There may be **erythema of the palms** (**249**) similar to that seen in pregnancy, rheumatoid arthritis and liver disease.

248

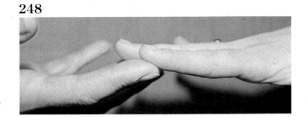

249

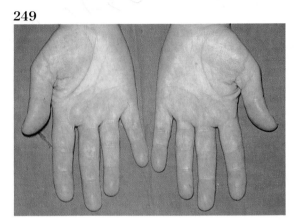

The **pulse** is rapid and forceful and in the elderly, atrial fibrillation may be present (**250**).

250

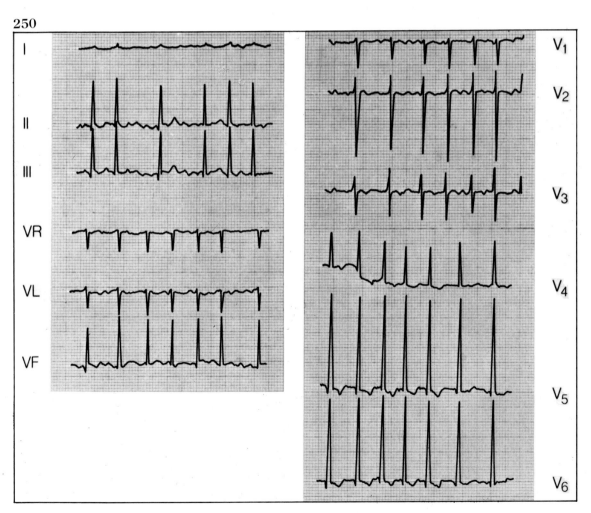

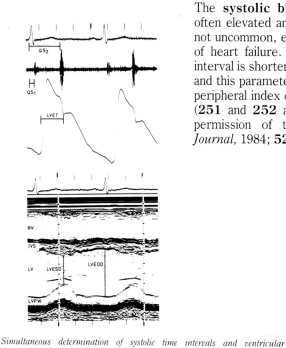

The **systolic blood pressure** is often elevated and ankle oedema is not uncommon, even in the absence of heart failure. The systolic time interval is shortened (**251** and **252**) and this parameter can be used as a peripheral index of thyroid function. (**251** and **252** are reproduced by permission of the *British Heart Journal*, 1984; **52**: 215–222.)

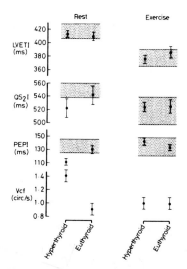

Simultaneous determination of systolic time intervals and ventricular dimensions from combined echophonocardiography. LVET, left ventricular ejection time; QS$_1$, electromechanical delay; PEP, pre-ejection period; ICT, isovolumetric contraction time; LVEDD/LVESD, left ventricular end diastolic/end systolic dimensions; RV, right ventricle; IVS, interventricular septum; LV, left ventricle; LVPW, left ventricular posterior wall. PEP = QS$_2$–LVET; ICT = PEP–QS$_1$.

Mean (SEM) values of systolic time interval and velocity of circumferential shortening of the left ventricle in 15 hyperthyroid patients and the same patients euthyroid at rest and during isometric exercise before and after autonomic blockade. Hatched areas denote predicted values (1 SD) for normal subjects. LVETI, left ventricular ejection time index; QS$_2$ I, electromechanical systole index; PEPI, pre-ejection period index; Vcf, velocity of circumferential fibre shortening.

Weight loss may be apparent (**253**) and partial lipodystrophy affecting the face in particular is an uncommon association (**254**). Proximal myopathy (**255**) is a rare presenting feature and causes difficulty in climbing stairs. Even rarer is Basedow's paraparesis, presenting as reversible pyramidal tract lesions. Splenomegaly and lymphadenopathy are occasionally seen.

253

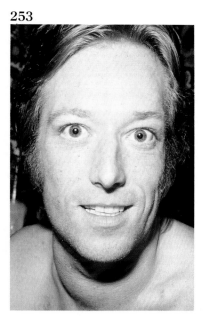

254

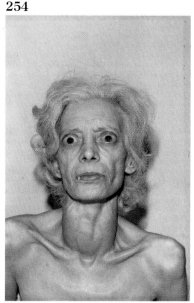

255

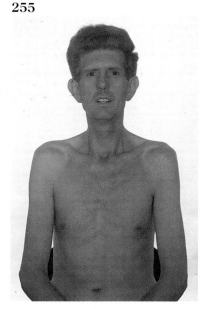

Transplacental passage of stimulating thyrotrophin receptor antibodies is responsible for the rare syndrome of transient neonatal hyperthyroidism (**256** and **257**). Mothers of such children have Graves' disease, usually with eye signs (**258**) and not infrequently with localised myxoedema. The condition must be differentiated from early onset Graves' disease, seen here in a boy aged 10 months (**259**). Graves' disease in children (**260**) usually persists for many years. Blocking of the thyrotrophin receptors has recently been recognised as a cause of transient neonatal hypothyroidism (**261**). In such cases the mother usually suffers from myxoedema or Hashimoto's disease and several siblings may be affected.

256

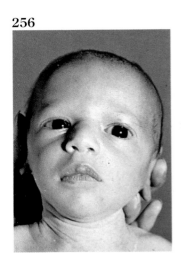

257

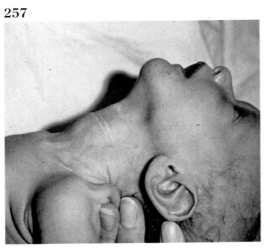

258

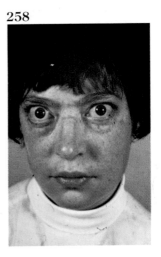

259

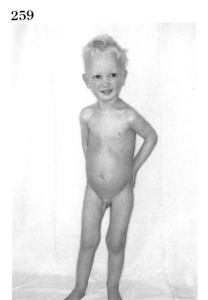

260

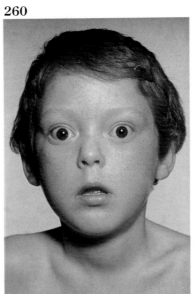

261

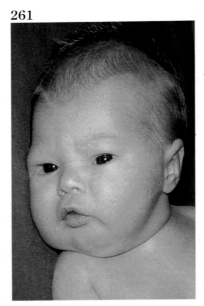

Eye signs

The eye signs of Graves' disease consist of varying combinations of the following:

- Exophthalmos (proptosis)
- Upper lid retraction
- Ptosis (rare)
- Periorbital swelling
- Ophthalmoplegia
- Chemosis, superficial punctate keratitis, conjunctivitis, injection over the insertion of the orbital muscles
- Congestive ophthalmopathy

Exophthalmos results from enlargement of muscles and fat within the orbit causing protrusion of the globe. It is usually present when sclera is visible between the lower lid and the margin of the cornea (**262**), but this sign may also occur in patients with familial shortness of the lower lids (**263**). This sign is most marked laterally and inspection of previous photographs reveals it as a permanent feature. The exophthalmos can be measured using a Hertel exophthalmometer (**264**). When the distance from the lateral orbital margin to the front of the cornea exceeds 18mm, exophthalmos is present (**265**).

262

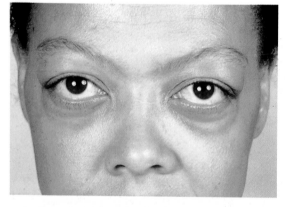

263

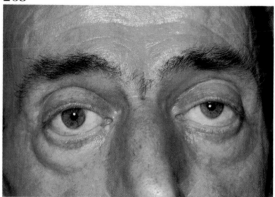

264

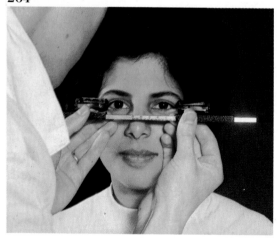

265

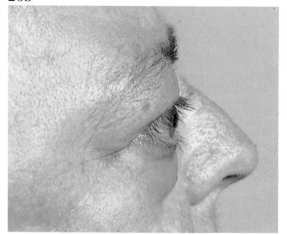

Exophthalmos is usually bilateral in hyperthyroid Graves' disease but is often unilateral in the ophthalmic form in which the patient is not, and never has been hyperthyroid (**266**). The asymmetry of the eyes in Graves' disease rarely exceeds 5mm: asymmetry in excess of this should suggest the possibility of a space-occupying lesion. **267** shows proptosis caused by an orbital tumour and its subsequent demonstration by computerised axial tomography (CT scan). **268** and **269** show the characteristic appearance of the orbit on CT scan in a patient with Graves' ophthalmopathy with enlarged muscles.

266

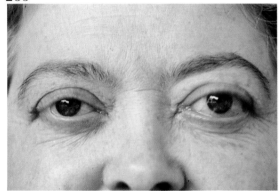

267

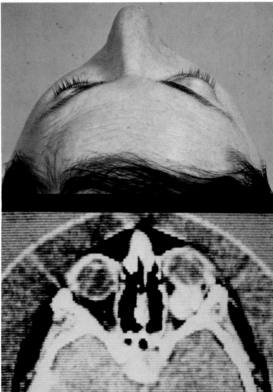

268

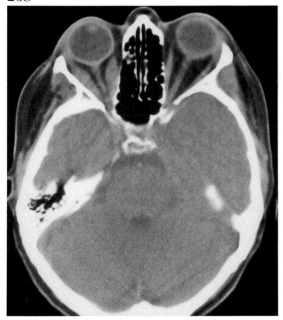

269

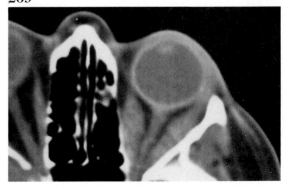

Other causes of unilateral proptosis include:

- Lymphoma of the orbit, occasionally bilateral, which often leads to deviation of the ocular axes (**270**)

- Pseudotumour of the orbit in which swelling of the lids may be prominent (**271** to **273**). The CT scan differs clearly from that seen in Graves' disease

- Caroticocavernous fistula in which the conjunctiva is injected and in which a vascular murmur may be heard over the globe (**274** and **275**)

- Mucocoele (**276**) arising from the frontal sinus, when radiographs reveal a break in the continuity of the bone (**277** and **278**). The mucocoele can be demonstrated by CT scan (**279**)

- Myopia when the globe itself is enlarged. **280** shows the concomitant strabismus of the amblyopic eye, as well as a cataract

- Orbital tendinitis is a rare cause of painful exophthalmos and ophthalmoplegia (**281**) characterised by intermittent pain and swelling and an atypical pattern of strabismus

- Dacryoadenitis is a rare inflammatory cause of proptosis (**282**)

270

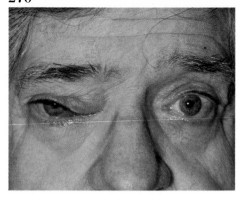

271

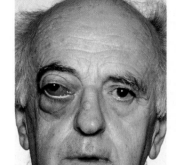

272

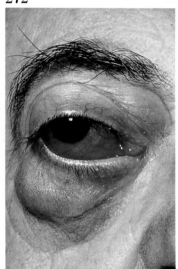

273

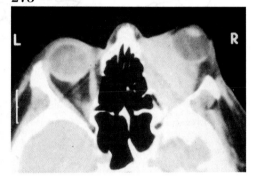

274

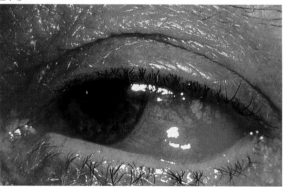

275

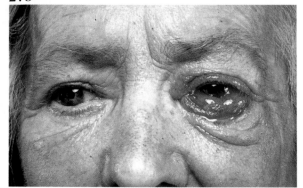

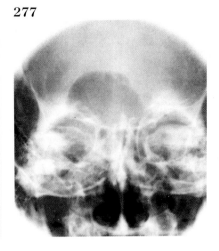

276

277

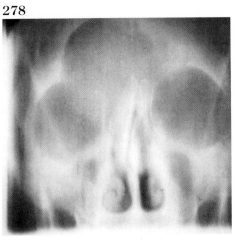

278

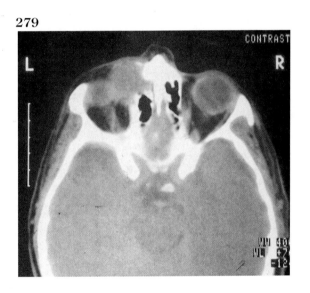

279

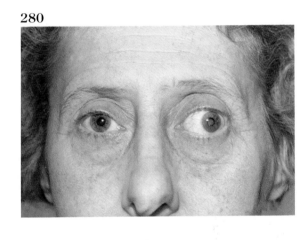

280

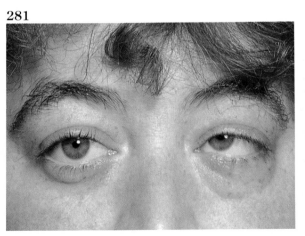

281

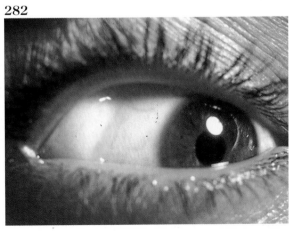

282

Lid retraction. This is a common eye sign in Graves' disease, recognised when sclera is visible between the lower margin of the upper lid and the cornea in the relaxed position of forward gaze (**283**). Minor degrees of lid retraction, insufficient to reveal the sclera, are best termed lid elevation (**284**). Severe lid retraction may lead to inadequate corneal coverage, particularly during the night, and is complicated by exposure keratitis (**285**). Swelling and overhanging of the upper lid may obscure the lid retraction (**286**). Lid retraction in hyperthyroid Graves' disease is usually bilateral (**287**), but unilateral retraction is quite common in the ophthalmic form (**288**). Lid retraction must be distinguished from elevation of the upper lids in an anxious patient who stares. It may also be seen in patients with lesions of the upper brain stem. **289** shows bilateral lid retraction in a patient with a vascular lesion of the brain stem: note the absence of other features of Graves' disease. **290** shows lid retraction in a patient with a brain stem glioma related to neurofibromatosis (**291**).

283

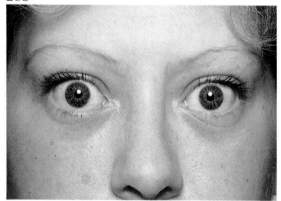

284

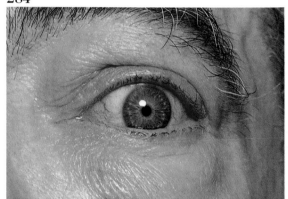

285

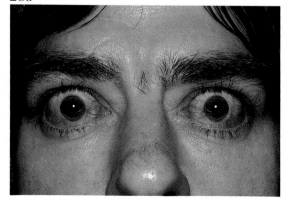

286

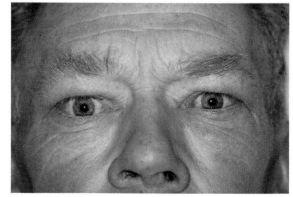

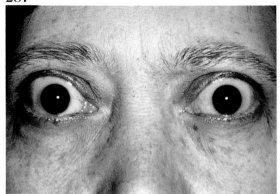

287

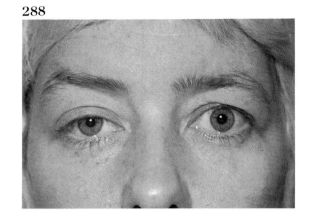

288

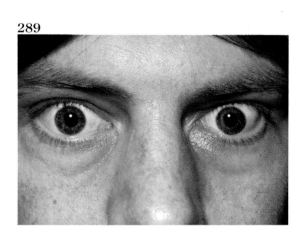

289

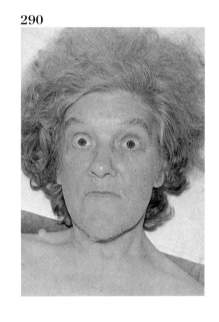

290

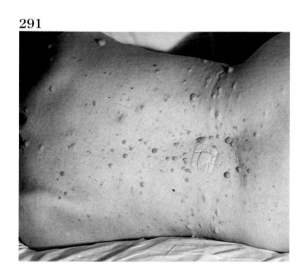

291

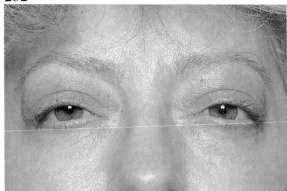

292

Ptosis. This rare sign of Graves' disease may be bilateral (**292**) or unilateral (**293** and **294**) and must always be differentiated from myasthenia gravis (**295**) by an edrophonium test.

293

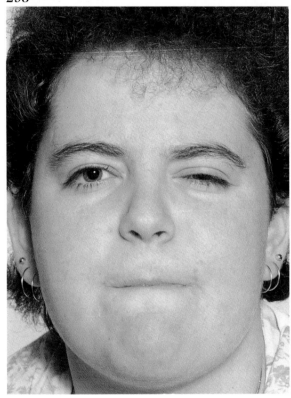

294

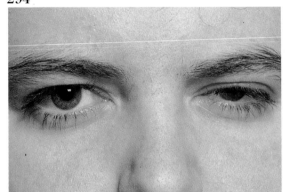

295

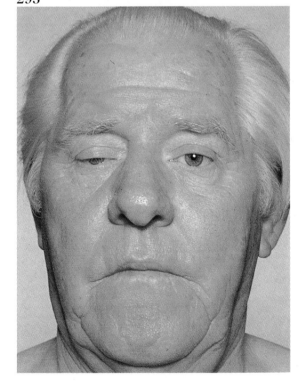

Periorbital swelling. This may give a slightly erythematous, oedematous appearance particularly affecting the upper lids (**296**) or, in association with exophthalmos, may be caused by bulging of the orbital contents through the natural hiatuses of the anterior orbital septum (**297**), most obvious medially. The latter appearance can be seen in any space-occupying lesion affecting the orbit. The swelling may be unilateral (**298**) or bilateral. The periorbital swelling of hypothyroidism (**299**) may resemble that of Graves' disease. Treatment of Graves' disease may lead to hypothyroidism when the periorbital swelling of both conditions is combined (**300**). Allergic reactions or angio-oedema affecting the eyelids can sometimes simulate Graves' disease (**301**).

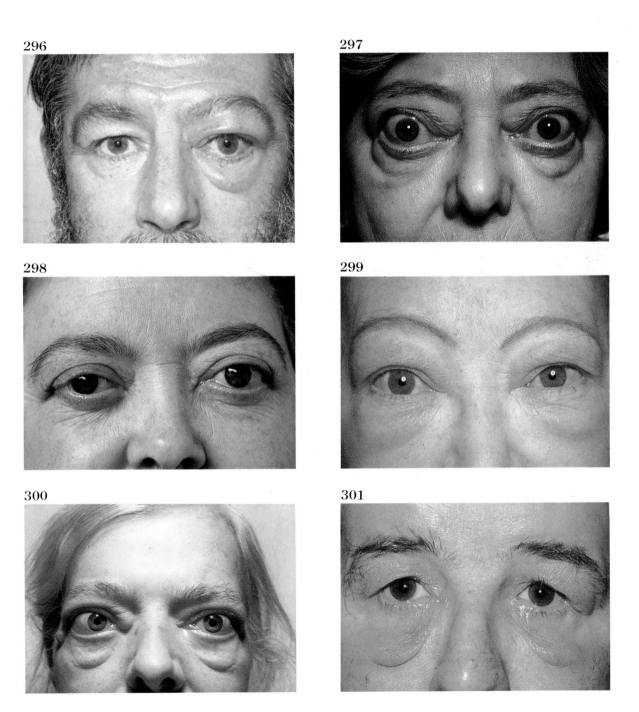

296

297

298

299

300

301

Ophthalmoplegia. This is one of the more distressing eye signs of Graves' disease. The muscles are initially swollen, oedematous and infiltrated with mucopolysaccharides and lymphocytes, but later become fibrotic and contracted. The presence of ophthalmoplegia may be suspected by the manner in which the patient tilts her head backwards in an effort to obtain binocular vision. Ophthalmoplegia rarely occurs as an isolated sign and is almost invariably accompanied by other eye signs of Graves' disease (**302**). The disease affects ocular movements in a characteristic sequence: upward and outward gaze (**303**), upward and inward, lateral, medial and downward gaze in diminishing order of frequency. The upward and outward gaze palsy, the direction of movement determined by the superior rectus, is caused by tethering of muscles below the globe. Looking upwards causes the patient more than usual discomfort.

Ophthalmoplegia affecting upward gaze may be accompanied by the paralytic form of lid retraction, in which retraction of the upper lid is enhanced when the patient looks up (**304**) and is abolished when the patient looks down (**305**). This contrasts with the commoner spastic form of lid retraction which changes little with different directions of gaze.

Chemosis, superficial punctuate keratitis, conjunctivitis, injection over insertion of the orbital muscles. Chemosis may be mild, when it can be demonstrated by pressing the lower lid against the conjunctivae (**306**), or so severe that the oedematous conjunctiva prolapses between the lids (**307**). Superficial punctuate keratitis may affect the upper limbus of the cornea in patients whose lid retraction leads to corneal exposure at night. Corneal ulceration is a dangerous sign seen in congestive ophthalmopathy, causing pain or discomfort in the eyes with lacrimation, photophobia and blepharospasm (**308**). Varying degrees of conjunctivitis are common in Graves' disease, being responsible for the feeling of grittiness or soreness and lacrimation (**309** and **310**). Injection over the insertions of the extraocular muscles, usually the lateral rectus, may be a sign of impending deterioration (**311**).

302

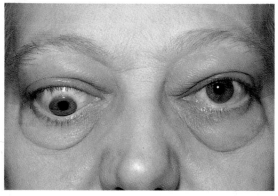

303

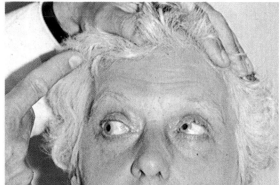

304

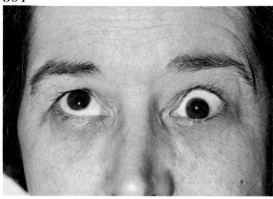

305

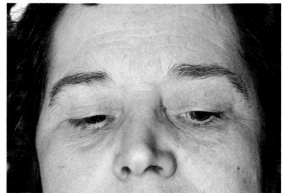

306

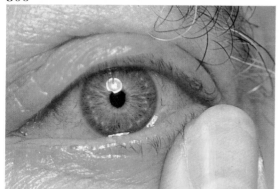

307

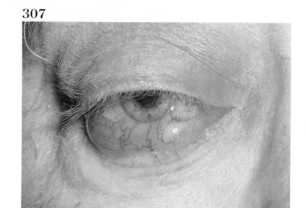

308

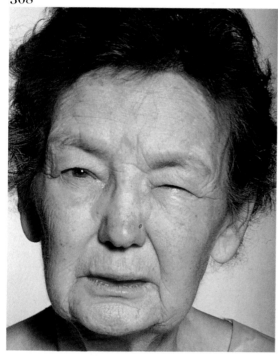

309

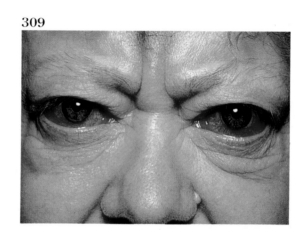

310

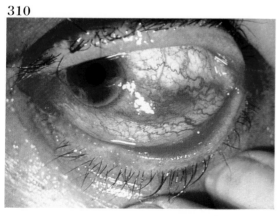

311

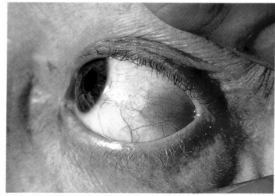

Congestive ophthalmopathy. This term has replaced 'malignant exophthalmos' as the condition is not malignant and often exophthalmos is absent. The eyes are inflamed and swollen, chemosis is invariable and the conjunctiva and swollen medial caruncles may prolapse between the lids (**312** and **313**). Periorbital oedema is usually marked and ophthalmoplegia is almost invariably present, whereas the more typical eye signs of exophthalmos and lid retraction are often absent. Papilloedema is uncommon and the fundi, apart from venous congestion, may appear surprisingly normal. The major risk of congestive ophthalmopathy is loss of vision, for which there are several causes:

- Corneal exposure can lead to ulceration

- Glaucoma with raised intraocular pressure accentuated by looking upwards is not uncommon

- Optic nerve compression causes loss of visual acuity, defects in colour vision and field defects, responsive to steroid therapy (**314** and **315** show concentric field defects occurring in congestive ophthalmopathy and their subsequent improvement after steroid therapy)

- Macular oedema also effects visual acuity (**316**).

- Refractive errors from compression of the globe by the swollen orbital contents can be corrected by appropriate lenses and should not be mistaken for optic nerve compression

Localised myxoedema usually affects the pretibial region (**317**) or the top of the feet but occasionally the hands, face or shoulders may be involved. Involvement of atypical sites may be determined by local trauma, as shown in the Thai farmer in **318**, who carried water suspended in buckets from a pole across his shoulders. Typically the skin is thickened, non-tender, red and violaceous in colour, with coarse hairs and little pitting oedema (**319**). The skin is infiltrated with mucopolysaccharides.

312

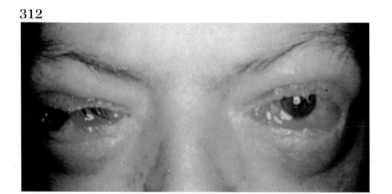

313

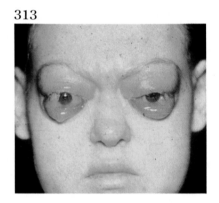

314

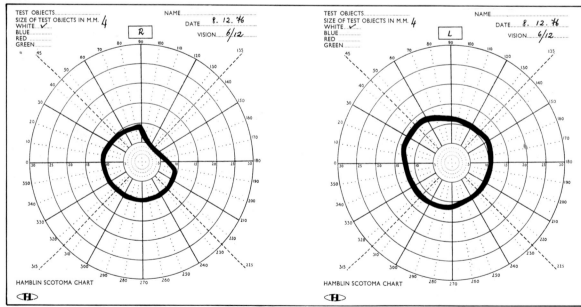

315

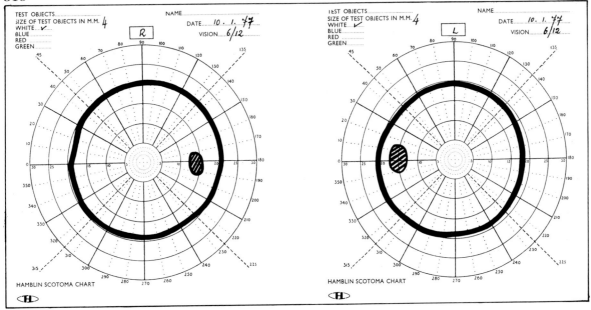

316

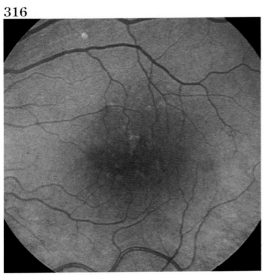

317

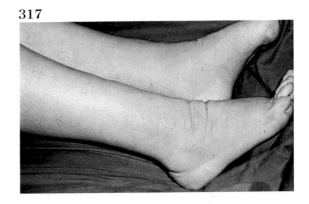

319

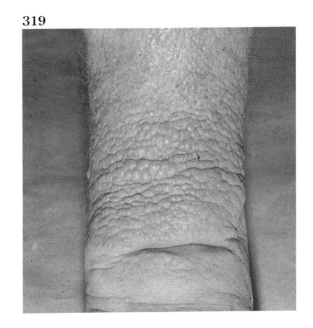

318

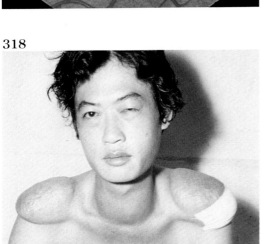

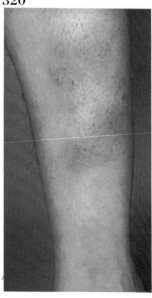

320

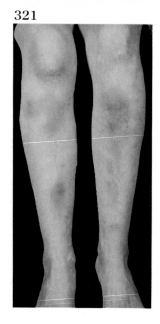

321

The underlying mechanism involved in the production of localised myxoedema is unknown, but the vast majority of patients have high circulating levels of TRAb. There are several forms of localised myxoedema, from the usual sheet form to a nodular variety (**320**) mimicking erythema nodosum (**321**) which should be easily distinguished because of its tenderness and the absence of other features of Graves' disease. Occasionally horny nodules develop on the dorsum of the feet or toes (**322** and **323**) which must be differentiated from pachyderma periostitis (**324**). Sometimes localised myxoedema resembles oedema of the legs or ankles but biopsy reveals typical histological changes.

Thyroid acropachy is considered on page 69.

322

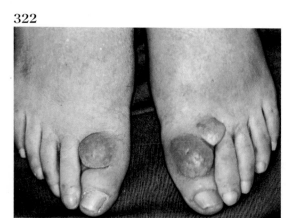

323

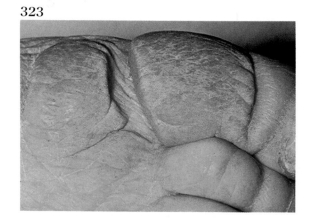

324

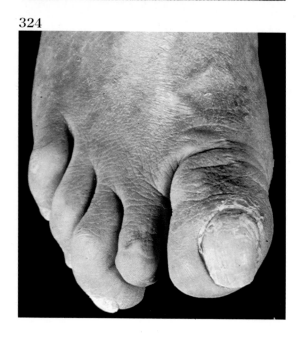

Other associated features of Graves' disease include:

Vitiligo (**325**) and its accompaniments (see later) are valuable cutaneous markers of organ-specific auto-immune disease. Gynecomastia is uncommon.

Splenomegaly is rare and other associated causes such as pernicious anaemia or iron deficiency should be sought.

Prominent jowls often accompanied by exophthalmos can produce a characteristic frog-face appearance in some patients (**326** and **327**).

Myasthenia gravis is a known but rare association of Graves' disease and can cause problems in diagnosis with the ophthalmic variety of Graves' (**328**).

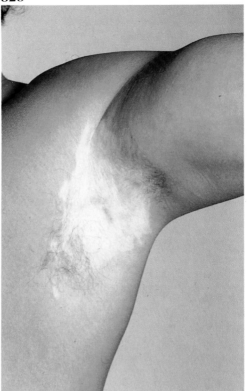

326

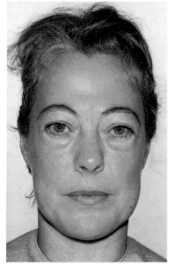

327

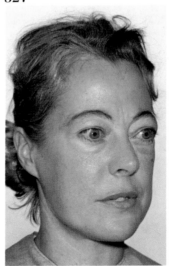

328

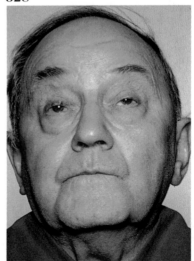

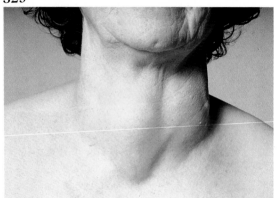

Toxic multinodular goitre

Toxic multinodular goitre is commoner in older patients (**329**) and in areas of iodine deficiency (**330**). Hyperthyroidism is readily precipitated by iodine ingestion (Jod–Basedow phenomenon) in a patient with a pre-existing nodular goitre (**331**). Eye signs are usually absent unless Graves' disease is superimposed on a pre-existing nodular goitre. Cardiovascular signs with atrial fibrillation and heart failure are common in these elderly patients (**332** and **333**). The thyroid scan shows a patchy uptake (**334**) and the ultrasound is characteristic (**335**).

330

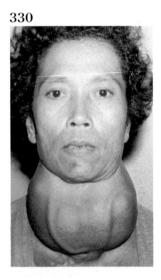

331

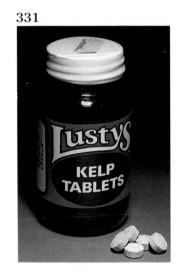

332

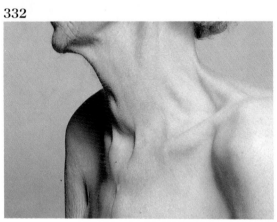

333

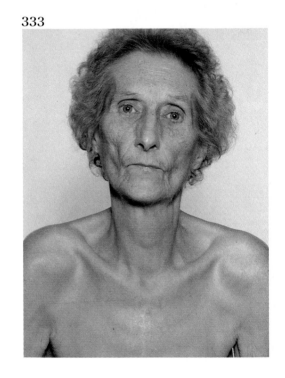

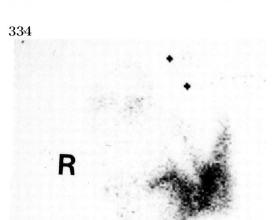

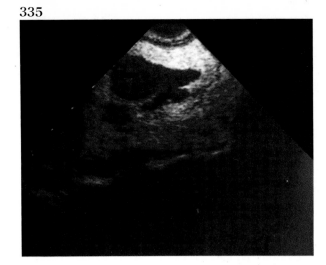

Toxic adenoma

Toxic adenoma (**336**) is also commoner in areas of iodine deficiency. Here one or more nodules function autonomously and cause hyperthyroidism. Occasionally nodules have autonomous function but do not produce enough thyroid hormone to cause hyperthyroidism, the so-called subclinical toxic adenoma. In such patients hyperthyroidism occurs when the nodule reaches a critical size, or if the patient is exposed to iodine. T_3 toxicosis is common in toxic adenoma, probably because of the lower intrathyroidal iodine pool. The thyroid scan shows a typical appearance (**337**) with suppression of the rest of the gland. Uptake by the nodule is not suppressed by triiodothyronine but TSH can increase uptake in the normal paranodular tissue. Autonomous nodules demonstrated by radioiodine are rarely malignant, but if technetium scanning is used, carcinomas may appear as hot nodules because they trap but do not organify the isotope.

336

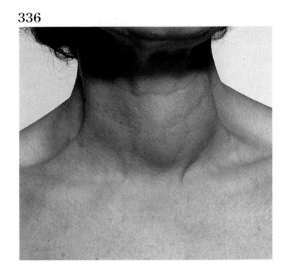

337

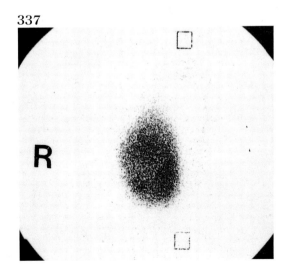

Hypothyroidism

Hypothyroidism is the clinical condition resulting from decreased circulating levels of free thyroid hormones, particularly free T_4 (fT_4). Factors involved in the control of TSH secretion are shown in **338**. Primary thyroid failure is characterised by decreased levels of f T_4 and increased circulating TSH. In pituitary hypothyroidism fT_4 is low and TSH low, normal or slightly raised. The raised level is caused by the production of abnormally glycosylated TSH with reduced biological activity as a result of deficiency of thyrotrophin-releasing hormone.

Primary thyroid failure can result from a wide variety of processes including:

- Autoimmune thyroid disease (AIT)
    Myxoedema
    Hashimoto's disease
    Post-partum thyroiditis

- Goitrogens

- Destructive therapy for hyperthyroidism or carcinoma
    Thyroidectomy
    Radioactive iodine

- Endemic iodine deficiency
    Endemic cretinism
    Endemic goitre

- Congenital defects
    Athyreosis, hypoplasia or ectopic thyroid
    Dyshormonogenesis

- Subacute de Quervain's thyroiditis

338

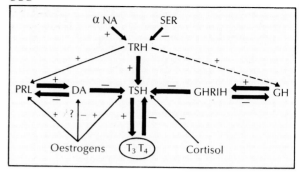

Autoimmune thyroid disease (AIT)

The autoimmune thyroid diseases are characterised by the presence of circulating thyroid antibodies, lymphocytic infiltration of the thyroid and variable alterations in thyroid function. They include the following conditions:

- Graves' disease (see above) with hyperthyroidism, ophthalmic Graves' disease
    Neonatal hyperthyroidism
    Neonatal hypothyroidism

- Myxoedema

- Hashimoto's disease

- Post-partum thyroiditis

- Lymphocytic thyroiditis

- Other associated conditions
    Vitiligo
    Halo naevi
    Leucotrichia
    Premature greying of the hair
    Alopecia areata

339

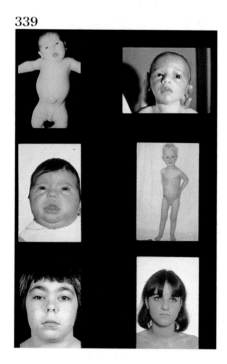

340

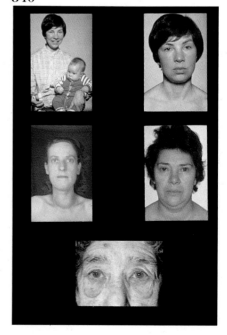

The spectrum of the different autoimmune diseases at different ages is shown in **339** and **340**. It ranges from intrauterine changes in thyroid function, to neonatal hyper- and hypothyroidism, juvenile hyper- and hypothyroidism, lymphocytic thyroiditis, silent thyroiditis, post-partum thyroiditis, Graves' disease, Hashimoto's disease and myxoedema.

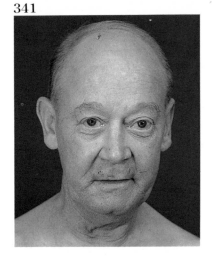

Autoimmune thyroid disease is one of the commonest organ-specific autoimmune diseases and is often associated with one of the following conditions:

- Diabetes mellitus
- Pernicious anaemia. **341** shows a man with previous Graves' disease, now with hypothyroidism and pernicious anaemia
- Addison's disease **342**. Some Addisonian patients have Schmidt's syndrome — the combination of permanent hypothyroidism and adrenal failure. Others have transient biochemical hypothyroidism
- Premature ovarian failure, often combined with Addison's disease
- Allergic alveolitis
- Renal tubular acidosis
- Rheumatoid arthritis, Sjögren's syndrome and myasthenia gravis
- Primary biliary cirrhosis and chronic active hepatitis

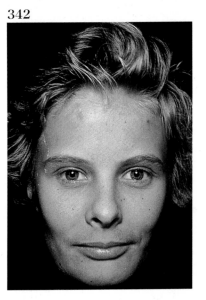

Hypothyroidism resulting from AIT may be associated with a goitre, when the term **Hashimoto's disease** is used, though some patients with Hashimoto's are euthyroid and in some hyperthyroidism may be present. The typical patient with Hashimoto's disease is a middle-aged woman with a diffuse, firm, finely nodular goitre who may be euthyroid or hypothyroid (**343**). Patients with **myxoedema** are again usually women, but older and are hypothyroid without thyroid enlargement (**344**).

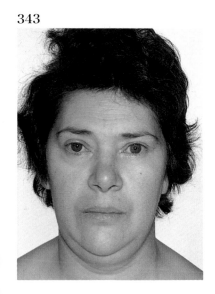

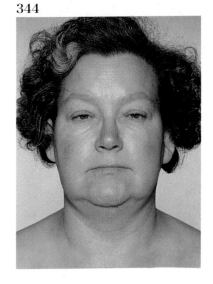

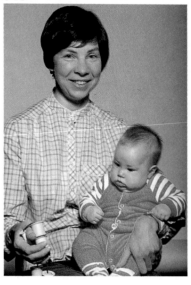

346

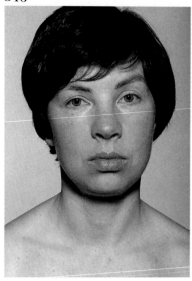

Post-partum thyroiditis (PPT) occurs in about 5 per cent of women three to six months after delivery. Women with pre-existing lymphocytic thyroiditis and microsomal antibodies are at risk of PPT. **345** shows a woman three months after delivery when she was well but had a small firm goitre. One month later she was symptomatically and biochemically hypothyroid (**346**). Asymptomatic hyperthyroidism commonly precedes the hypothyroidism which itself remits spontaneously in a few months in most cases.

347

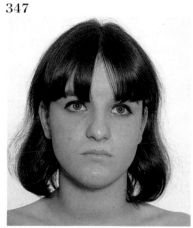

Lymphocytic thyroiditis is the term applied to patients, usually younger than those with Hashimoto's disease, with small goitres showing a lesser degree of lymphocytic infiltration and circulating thyroid antibodies (**347**). Some 10 per cent of young women have significant titres of microsomal antibodies. It is from this pool of patients that PPT and, in later life, Hashimoto's disease and myxoedema are largely derived.

348

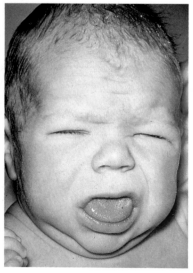

Neonatal hypothyroidism occurs in infants born to mothers with AIT, myxoedema, Hashimoto's disease or Graves' disease who have circulating antibodies which block the action of TSH on the thyroid (**348**). The disease is self-limiting and remits as the level of circulating antibodies falls.

Other associated conditions:

349

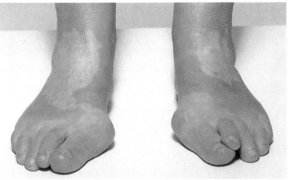

350

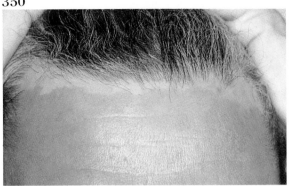

• Vitiligo, the patchy, almost symmetrical de-pigmentation of the skin surrounded by increased pigmentation (**349**), is a marker for all of the organ-specific autoimmune diseases (**350**).

• Halo naevi — where a pigmented naevus is surrounded by a depigmented halo (**351**) with ultimate disappearance of the naevus.

351

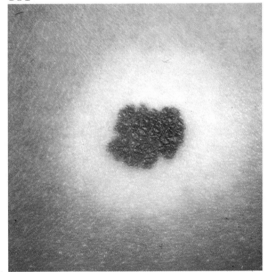

• Leucotrichia — white patches of hair affecting the eyelashes (**352**), body hair or scalp.

352

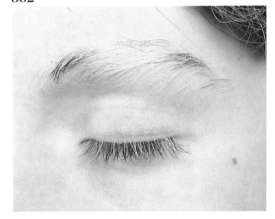

353

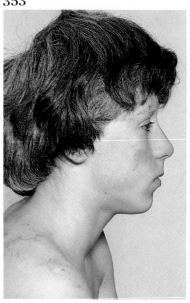

● Premature greying of the hair is seen characteristically in pernicious anaemia but also in AIT. **353** shows a 13-year-old boy with greying of the hair.

● Alopecia areata, the patchy loss of scalp hair (**354** and **355**) may be precipitated by emotional stress. Alopecia totalis may also be seen (**356**).

354

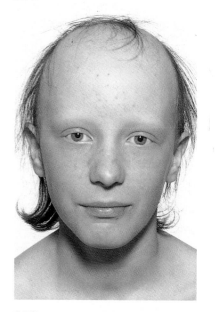

355

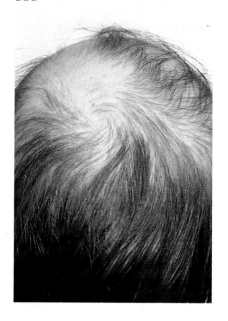

356

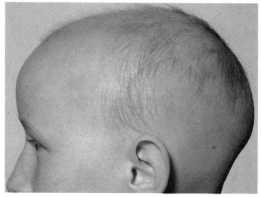

Goitrogens are a not uncommon cause of goitre with or without hypothyroidism. They differ from country to country. Cassava is a common goitrogen in areas of endemic iodine deficiency (**357**). Iodine from cough medicines, vitamin pills, X-ray contrast media or certain drugs such as amiodarone, are common goitrogens in the UK. **358** shows a man with asthma whose goitre resulted from an iodine-containing proprietary asthma medication.

357

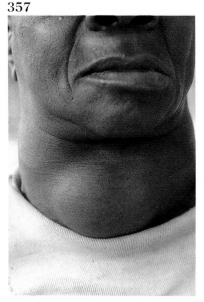

358

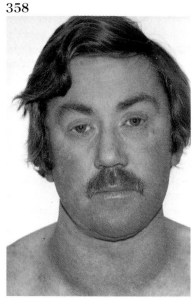

Destructive therapy to the thyroid is a common cause of hypothyroidism and may be suspected in patients with thyroidectomy scars or residual eye signs of Graves' disease (**359**).

359

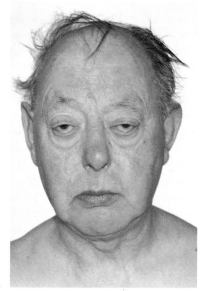

360

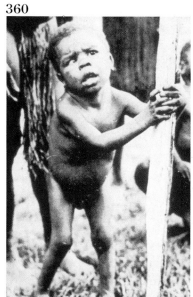

Endemic iodine deficiency affecting pregnant women can lead to neurologic endemic cretinism (**360** and **361**), or to endemic goitre (**362**) in the offspring with or without clinical and biochemical evidence of hypothyroidism.

361

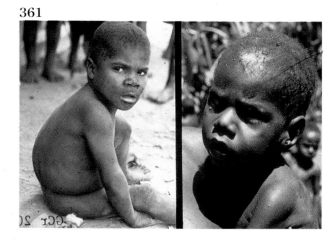

362

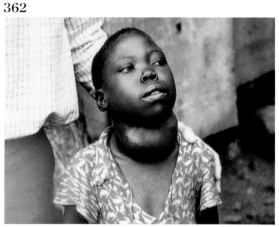

Ectopic thyroids are the commonest cause of neonatal hypothyroidism in most areas. The thyroid can be situated anywhere from the base of the tongue to its normal position. Before removing an ectopic thyroid it is important to ascertain by scanning whether there is thyroid tissue present in the normal position. **363** shows a child with an ectopic thyroid and the corresponding ^{123}I-scan (**364**). **365** shows a scan of an ectopic sublingual thyroid without normal thyroid tissue. By contrast **366** and **367** show a thyroglossal cyst and the corresponding scan showing no uptake in the thyroglossal cyst, but all of the uptake in the normal thyroid.

363

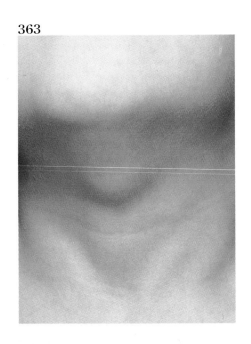

364

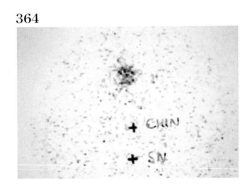

365

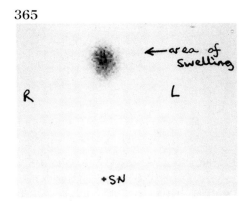

366

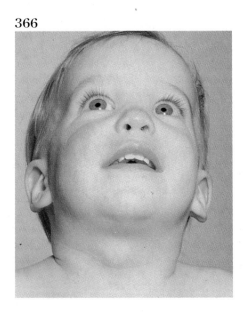

367

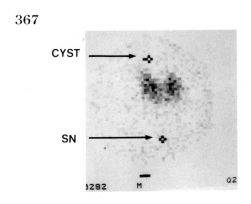

368 illustrates a highly placed goitre caused by autoimmune thyroiditis mimicking a thyroglossal cyst.

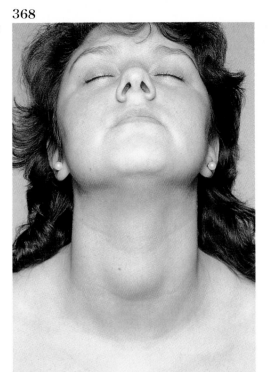

An ectopic thyroid may fail at any time from in utero to old age. The long-standing thyroid failure which sometimes results can lead to feedback thyrotroph hyperplasia with enlargement of the pituitary fossa (**369**).

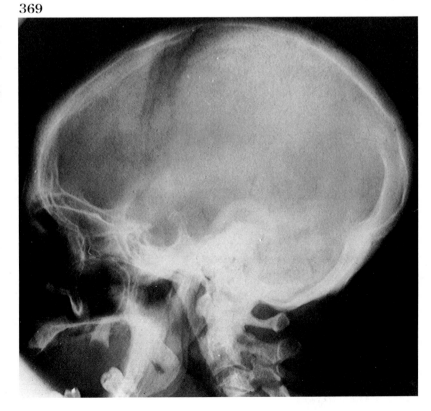

Athyreosis or hypoplasia of the thyroid are common causes of neonatal hypothyroidism (**370**), which can be recognised by thyroid scanning. Athyreotic infants almost invariably have retarded bone age, as shown in **371**, when the epiphyses normally present in utero are absent or dysgenetic. The bony changes of cretinism include widening of the epiphyseal line, deformed epiphyses, abnormal bone texture and irregularity of the metaphyses. Most of these features are shown in the hand radiographs of a 12-year-old cretin (**372**). With modern screening programmes elderly cretinism (**373**) should now be a disease of the past.

370

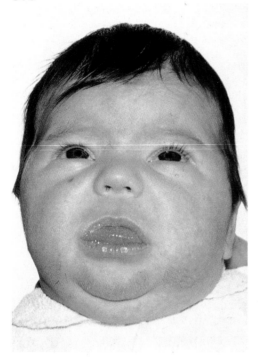

371

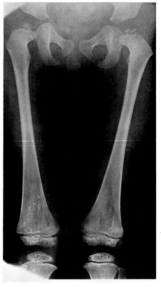

373

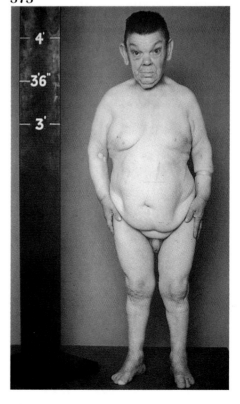

372

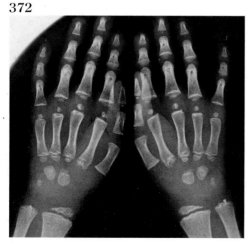

Dyshormonogenesis should be suspected in children with goitres with or without evidence of a family history of thyroid disease (**374**). There are many enzyme defects which can cause thyroid disease, the organification process being most commonly affected, resulting in Pendred's syndrome of goitre, hypothyroidism, deaf mutism and mental retardation in some cases (**375**). The condition is easily diagnosed by the perchlorate discharge test, where administration of potassium perchlorate leads to discharge of non-organically bound iodine from the thyroid. Certain types of goitre are associated with calcification visible on radiographs of the neck (**376**).

374

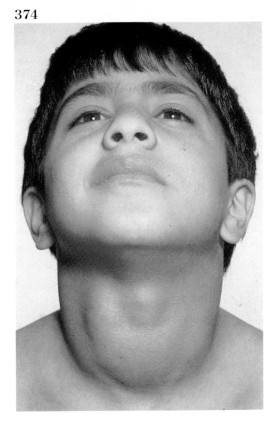

375

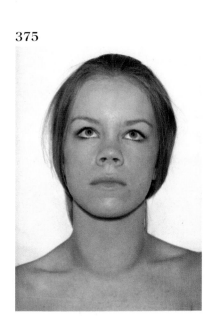

376

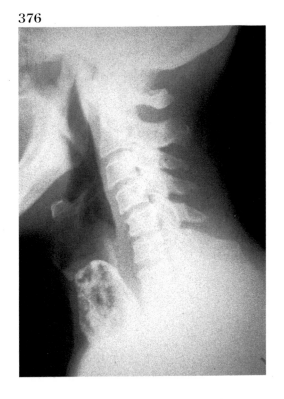

377

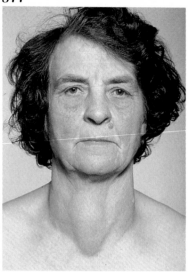

Subacute de Quervain's thyroiditis, a virally mediated inflammation of the thyroid, results in an initial increase in thyroid function. Later development of hypothyroidism is rare. The thyroid is diffusely enlarged, firm and painful (**377**). Systemic upset is common. The radioiodine uptake is suppressed.

378

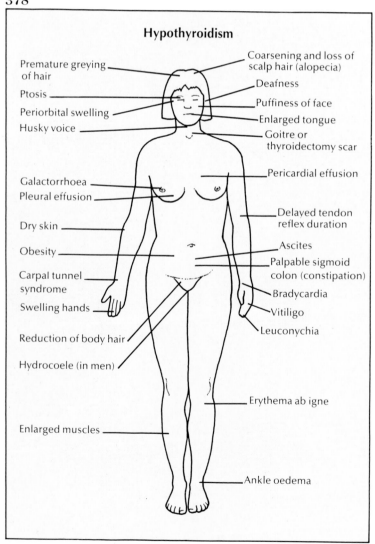

Hypothyroidism

Premature greying of hair

Ptosis

Periorbital swelling

Husky voice

Galactorrhoea

Pleural effusion

Dry skin

Obesity

Carpal tunnel syndrome

Swelling hands

Reduction of body hair

Hydrocoele (in men)

Enlarged muscles

Coarsening and loss of scalp hair (alopecia)

Deafness

Puffiness of face

Enlarged tongue

Goitre or thyroidectomy scar

Pericardial effusion

Delayed tendon reflex duration

Ascites

Palpable sigmoid colon (constipation)

Bradycardia

Vitiligo

Leuconychia

Erythema ab igne

Ankle oedema

Clinical features of hypothyroidism

The characteristic clinical features of hypothyroidism are shown in **378**. They include the following:

- Coarsening and loss of scalp hair (**379**)

379

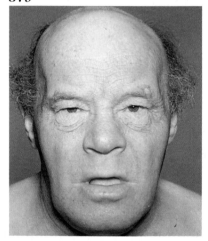

- Puffiness of the face with peri-orbital swelling which may be mild or gross (**380**) and which improves with therapy (**381** and **382**)

380

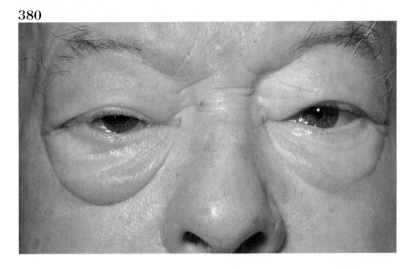

381

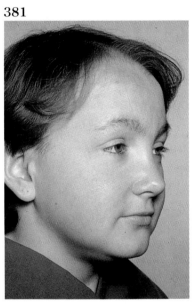

382

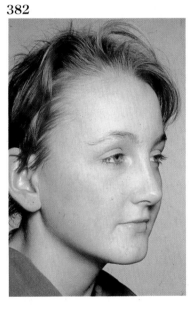

- Goitre, a thyroidectomy scar (**383**) or eye signs of Graves' disease indicating the presence of underlying thyroid disease

383

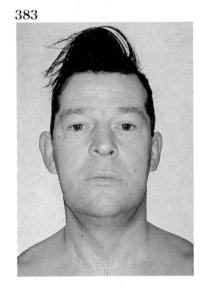

384

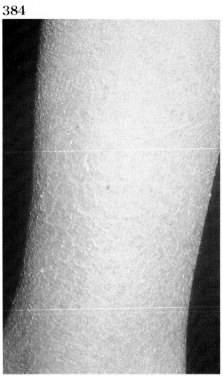

● Dryness of the skin (**384**), leuconychia (**385**), also seen in chronic liver disease, erythema ab igne (**386**), reduced body hair and yellow palms from carotenaemia (**387**)

385

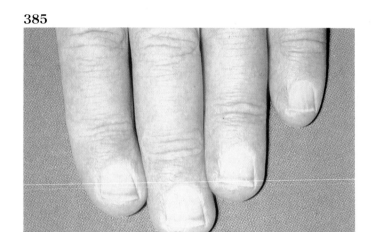

386

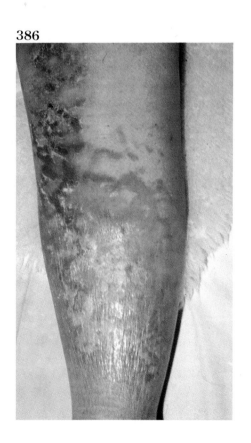

387

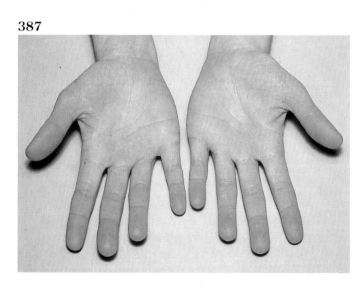

- Prolonged relaxation of the tendon reflexes, a feature of overt hypothyroidism, can be demonstrated clinically by gentle percussion of the biceps tendon, and measured as the Achilles tendon reflex duration (ATRD). The ATRDs of a euthyroid and hypothyroid subject are shown in **388**. Muscle enlargement and stiffness are rare accompaniments (Hoffman's syndrome) shown in **389**

388

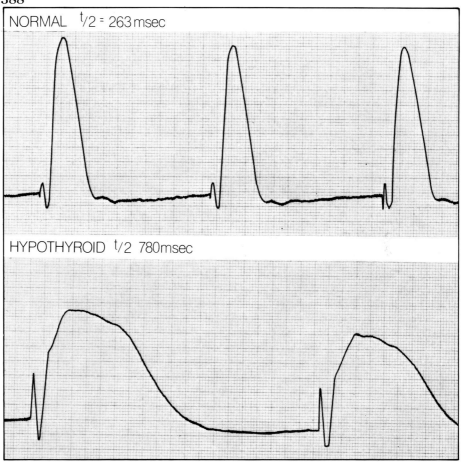

NORMAL $^t/2 = 263$ msec

HYPOTHYROID $^t/2$ 780msec

389

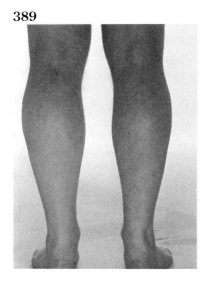

390

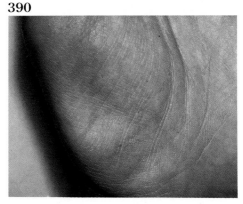

- Peripheral neuropathy or nerve entrapment syndromes, especially the carpal tunnel syndrome, which may lead to wasting of the thenar eminence (**390**)

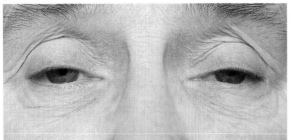

391

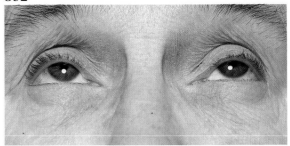

392

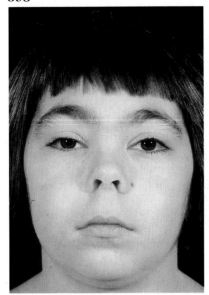

393

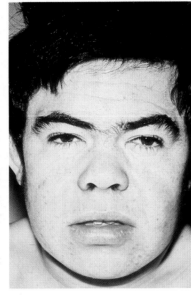

394

- Ptosis may be marked (**391** and **392**)

- Juvenile hypothyroidism (**393**) often presents with failure of growth but can be mimicked by other metabolic disorders such as Hurler's syndrome (**394**)

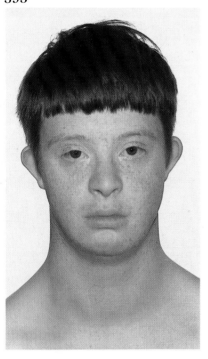

395

- Down's syndrome may be complicated by goitre and/or hypothyroidism caused by autoimmune thyroid disease (**395**)

- Body cavity effusions may lead to:

Pericardial effusion causing apparent cardiac enlargement, best demonstrated by echocardiography. **396** shows a two-dimensional echocardiogram in a patient with myxoedema showing a pericardial effusion (PE) anteriorly and posteriorly, RV = right ventricle, LV = left ventricle, IVS = inter-ventricular septum. **397** shows a standard echo of a pericardial effusion (1 = pericardial effusion, 2 = right ventricle, 3 = left ventricle, 4 = aorta, 5 = left atrium). **398** shows a pericardial effusion and **399** its resolution after thyroxine

Pleural effusions

Ascites (**400**)

Uveal effusions seen on fundoscopy (**401**) which impair vision and which can be demonstrated by ultrasound

Middle and inner ear effusions contribute to the deafness, dizziness and sometimes true vertigo seen in hypothyroidism

Hydrocoeles may be seen which remit with treatment of hypothyroidism

Joint effusions are uncommon

396

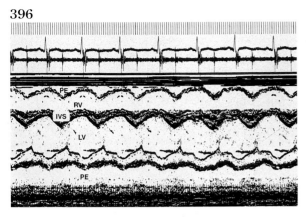

397

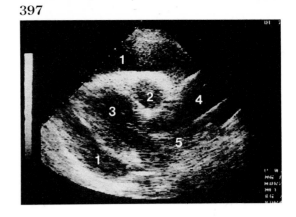

398

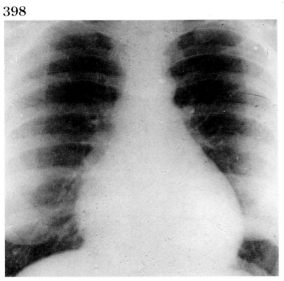

399

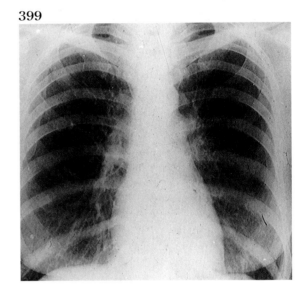

400

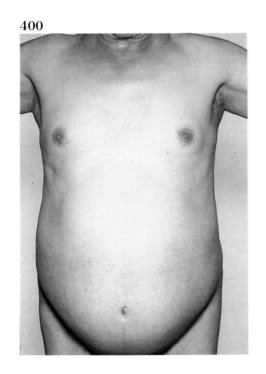

401

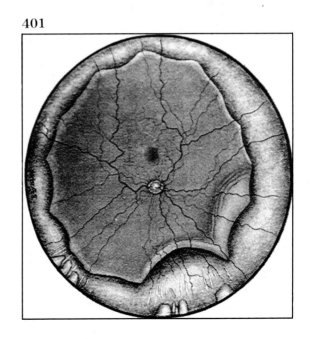

402

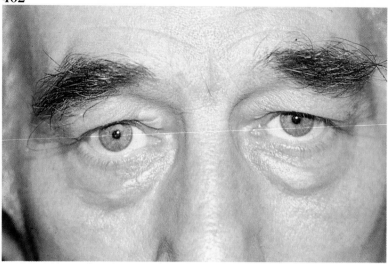

● Xanthelasma (**402**) is common in hypothyroidism even in the absence of lipid abnormalities

403

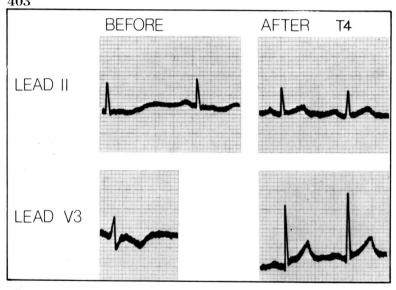

BEFORE   AFTER   T4

LEAD II

LEAD V3

● Electrocardiographic (ECG) changes of hypothyroidism may mimic ischaemic heart disease or hypertension. They consist of variable bradycardia, low voltage P and R waves and T inversion (**403**, **404** and **405**) which rapidly resolve with therapy

● Oedema of the ankles is sometimes striking and may take time to resolve with therapy

404

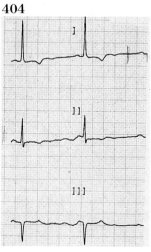

405

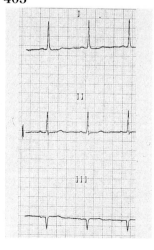

Hypothyroidism varies in severity from overt, which is easily recognisable clinically and biochemically, with a low fT$_4$ and markedly raised TSH (**406**), to mild with non-specific clinical features (**407**), and a border-line low or low normal fT$_4$ but slightly raised TSH. Differentiation between mild and subclinical hypo-thyroidism can be difficult or even impossible without a therapeutic trial of thyroid hormone.

406

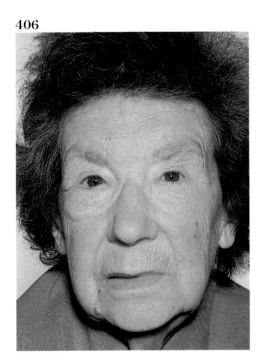

407

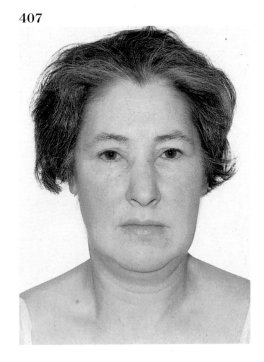

Goitre

Enlargement of the thyroid gland is referred to as a goitre. The problem facing the clinician when a patient complains of a swelling in the neck is to decide whether the thyroid is enlarged or not. A 'pseudo-goitre' usually results from a pad of fat over the front of the neck (**408**). The thyroid is rarely palpable in a normal man. In many thin women a normal thyroid can be felt. Observer variation in assessment of thyroid size is considerable, and it may be difficult to decide whether the patient has an easily palpable normal gland or a small goitre.

408

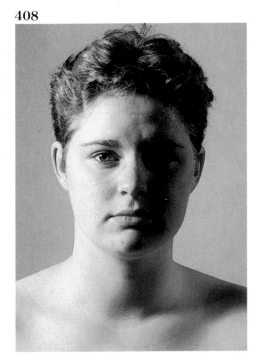

Classification of thyroid size and condition
Various classifications of thyroid size can be used but
in routine clinical practice goitres are best defined as:

- Small — palpable but not visible unless the neck
is very thin

- Moderate — thyroid visible but not large (**409**)

- Large — an obvious goitre which causes a definite
increase in neck circumference (**410**)

In addition to their size, goitres should be described
as diffuse (**411**) as seen in Graves' disease, multinodular (**412**) and or as a single nodule. The consistency
should be described as soft, normal, firm as in AIT, or
hard as in a carcinoma. One should always listen over
a thyroid for a vascular murmur which is almost
diagnostic of hyperthyroidism.

409

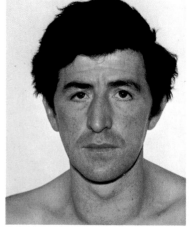

410

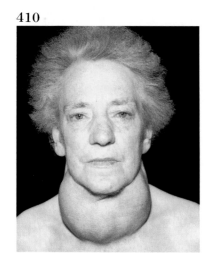

411

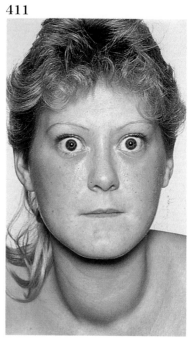

412

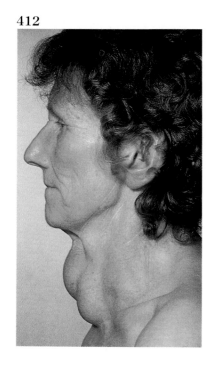

Prevalence of goitre varies in different parts of the world. In severely iodine-deficient areas goitres may affect 90 per cent of the population (**413** and **414**).

413

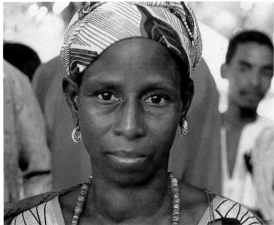

414

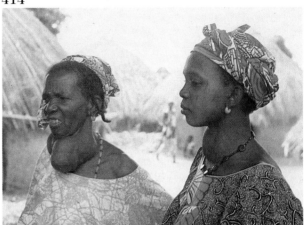

Types of goitre These are similar to the causes of hypothyroidism and include:

- Simple non-toxic goitre
- Endemic goitre
- Autoimmune thyroid disease
- Drug-induced goitre

- Dyshormonogenesis
- Ectopic thyroid
- Thyroid nodules and neoplasms

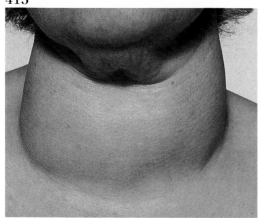

415

Simple non-toxic goitre. The term 'simple goitre' is used to describe thyroid enlargement without disturbance of thyroid function for which no obvious cause can be found. Some may be the result of previous iodine deficiency. Most goitres, which usually occur in women, fall into this category in the UK. Treatment is rarely required unless they are cosmetically disfiguring (**415**), cause pressure effects e.g. tracheal compression (**416**) or raise the suspicion of malignancy. In younger patients the thyroid is more likely to be generally enlarged (**417**) whereas nodules may be visible (**418**) in the older age group. **419** shows a scan of a nodular goitre. Patients with nodular goitres are at risk for the development of hyperthyroidism, particularly after iodine administration. The patchy uptake of iodine is well shown by autoradiography (**420**).

416

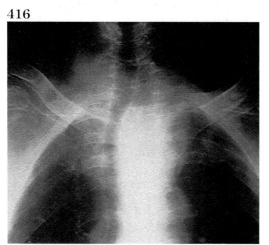

417

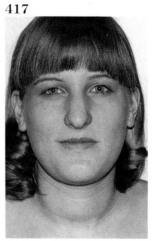

418

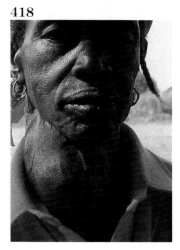

419

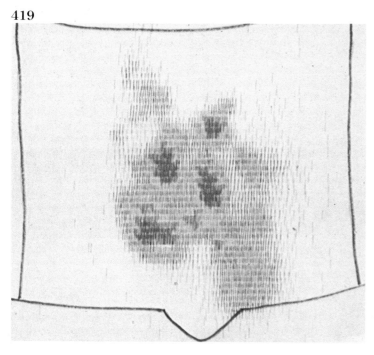

420

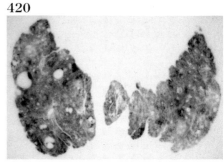

Retrosternal goitres can cause local pressure effects. Pressure on the veins can cause a superior mediastinal syndrome (**421**). Infra-red photography (**422**) and venography reveal the dilated veins (**423**). The mass is visible radiographically in the upper mediastinum (**424**), often causing tracheal displacement or narrowing (**425**) or oesophageal deviation, which can be seen on barium swallow (**426**). Scanning confirms the presence of thyroid tissue in an abnormally low position (**427**).

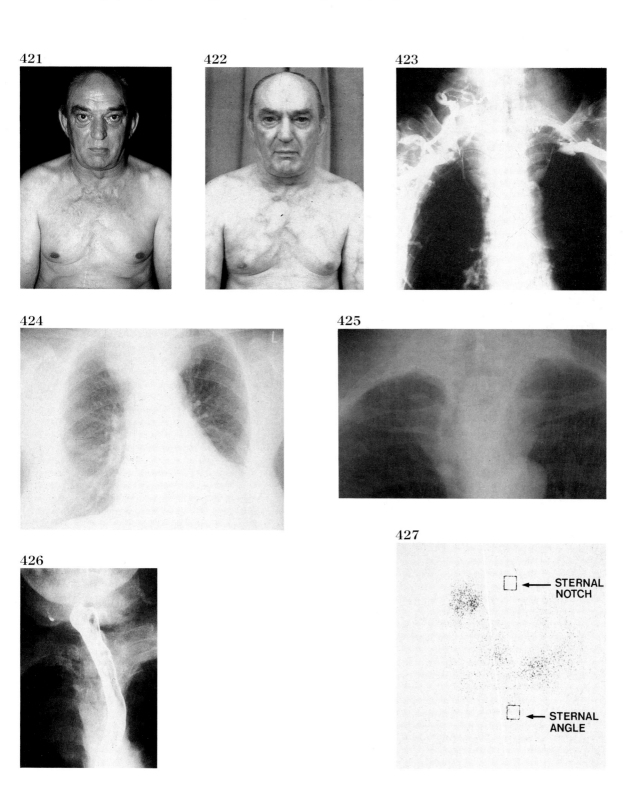

421

422

423

424

425

426

427

STERNAL NOTCH

STERNAL ANGLE

428

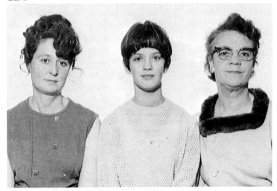

Endemic goitres are common in areas of severe and moderate iodine deficiency. Hypothyroidism is uncommon unless the iodine deficiency is severe. Endemic cretinism can be prevented by iodination programmes.

Autoimmune thyroid disease (see pages 90 and 91) is a common cause of thyroid enlargement in the UK. The goitre is usually small or moderate in size, diffusely enlarged, firm and finely nodular, often with a palpable pyramidal lobe. Several generations may be affected. 428 shows a girl with Hashimoto's disease, her mother with Graves' disease and her grandmother with myxoedema.

429

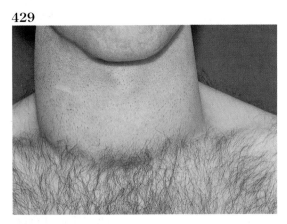

Drug-induced goitres are generally soft and diffusely enlarged. They show the sex preponderance of the underlying disease rather than the usual female preponderance of simple goitre. Hypothyroidism may be present and both thyroid failure and goitre usually respond to drug withdrawal. A variety of drugs can be responsible but in the UK iodides are a common cause (429).

Dyshormonogenesis (see page 99). Goitres resulting from dyshormonogenesis are initially soft and diffuse (430) but later become nodular. Recurrence after thyroidectomy is the rule. This cause should be considered in all children with a goitre, particularly if there is a family history of goitre.

430

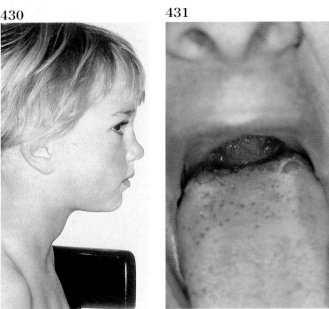

431

432

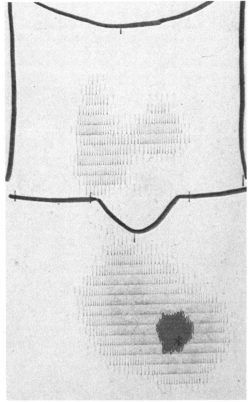

Ectopic thyroids (see pages 96 and 97) are found anywhere from the base of the tongue (431 — lingual thyroid) to the mediastinum (432 — scan of ectopic thyroid in the upper mediastinum).

Thyroid nodules and neoplasms

Thyroid nodules may be benign or malignant. Features which suggest malignancy include:

- Asymmetry (**433**)
- Unusual location of the swelling (**434**)
- Hardness
- Lymphadenopathy
- Increase in size. Rapid painful increase in size can be caused by haemorrhage into a nodule which can occasionally penetrate the capsule to give the appearance shown in **435** and **436**
- Hoarseness of the voice
- Fixation to skin and underlying tissues

433

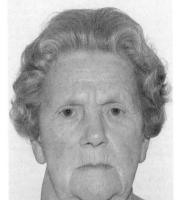

434

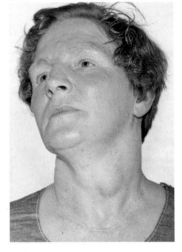

435

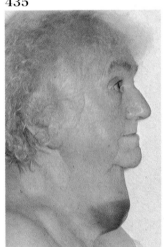

436

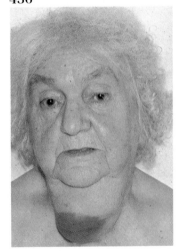

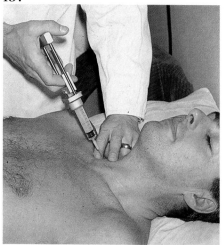

The most difficult diagnostic problem is the single thyroid nodule, about 10 per cent of which are malignant. The investigation of choice is now fine needle aspiration biopsy (**437**), which allows cytological recognition of follicular lesions (**438**), which always require surgical exploration, papillary carcinoma (**439** and **440**), thyroiditis or colloid nodules. Scanning of the nodule, using ^{123}I may be helpful (**441**). Functioning nodules are rarely malignant, whereas cold nodules may be malignant or represent a non-functioning adenoma, a cyst or an area of thyroiditis.

438

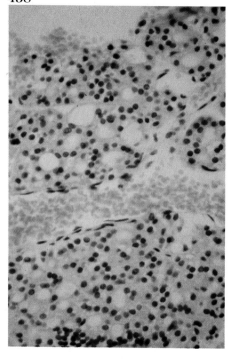

439

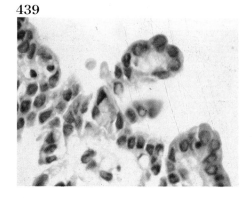

441

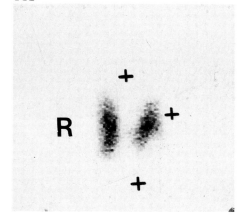

440

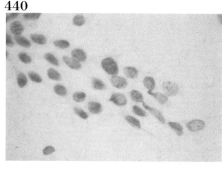

Ultrasound can help to identify a cyst. **442** shows a thyroid scan with a cyst shown in the lower pole of the left lobe. **443** shows a transverse view of a normal left thyroid lobe (L) at the level of the isthmus (I); the width of the lobe is measured between the trachea (T) and the carotid artery (C). **444** is a longitudinal view of the right thyroid lobe, demonstrating a hypoechoic solid mass 1.6 cm long. Small cysts (less than 4 cm in diameter) are usually benign. (**443** and **444** are reproduced by permission of the *New England Journal of Medicine*, 1987; **317**: 70–75.)

442

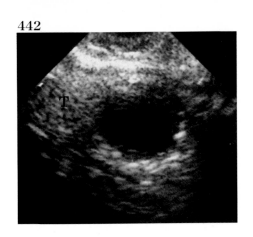

443

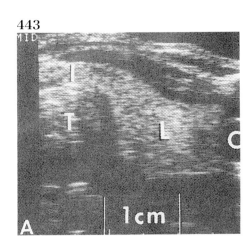

444

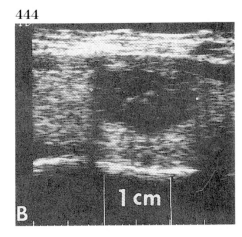

Carcinoma of the thyroid may be papillary. **445** shows typical lymph node invasion. **446** shows a ^{123}I scan of a papillary carcinoma with matching ultrasound (**447**).

445

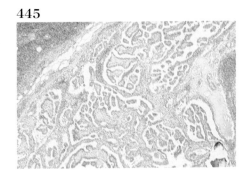

446

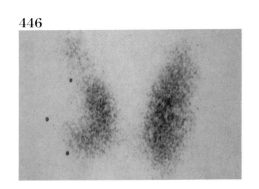

447

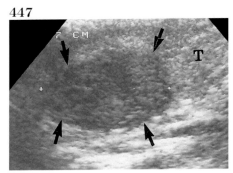

448

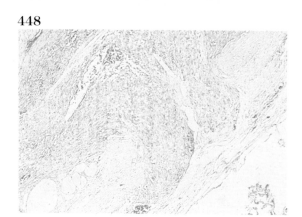

Follicular carcinomas often show invasion of the capsule of the gland (**448**). **449** shows a scan of a follicular carcinoma and the corresponding ultrasound (**450**). Medullary and anaplastic tumours of the thyroid are less common. Patients with carcinoma of the thyroid usually present with a thyroid nodule (features suggesting malignancy have already been listed above). Occasionally the presentation may be with metastases in lung (**451** shows multiple lung metastases), bone (**452** and **453**) or lymph nodes.

449

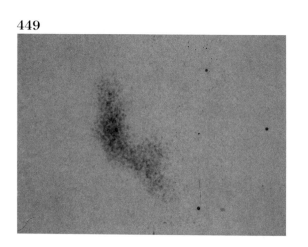

450

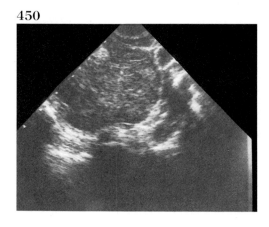

451

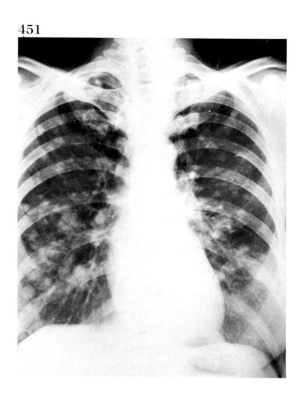

452

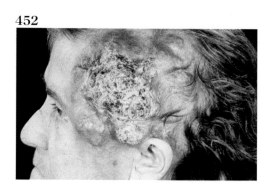

453

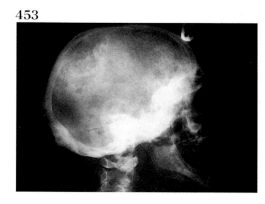

Medullary carcinoma of the thyroid is derived from the parafollicular or 'C cells' of the thyroid which produce calcitonin and often contain amyloid (**454**). This carcinoma may be sporadic or familial, when it may form part of the 'multiple endocrine neoplasia' syndrome (MEN). In MEN Type IIa it is associated with phaeochromocytoma and parathyroid adenoma. In MEN Type IIb medullary carcinoma is associated with:

- Marfanoid habitus (**455**)
- Mucosal neuromas of the lips (**456**), eyelids (**457**) and tongue (**458** and **459**)
- Proximal myopathy
- Ganglioneuromatosis of the bowel

Patients with this condition have a characteristic facial appearance.

455

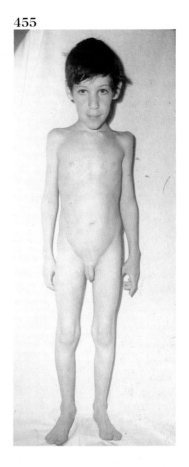

454

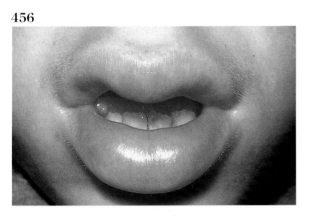

456

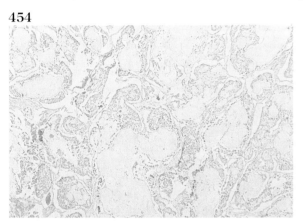

457

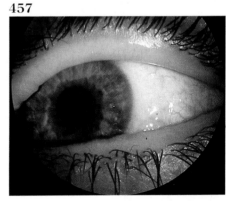

458

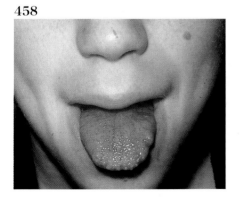

459

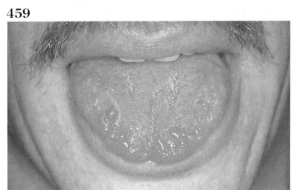

Chapter 4
Adrenal

Adrenal cortex

Introduction

The adrenal cortex secretes three groups of steroids, which are classified by their biological actions:

1. The glucocorticoids have major effects on glucose and protein metabolism, and a number of other metabolic actions. The principal naturally occurring glucocorticoid is cortisol, although a small amount of corticosterone is also secreted. Cortisol is the most potent glucocorticoid in man. Cortisone and 11-dehydrocorticosterone do not have intrinsic activity but are active after conversion to cortisol and corticosterone. The glucocorticoids are secreted by the zona fasciculata under the control of ACTH (corticotrophin).

2. The mineralocorticoids are steroids which have a major effect on electrolyte transport by epithelial cells leading to sodium conservation and potassium loss. The most potent of these is aldosterone, but 11-deoxycorticosterone (DOC), 18-hydroxy-DOC, and the glucocorticoids also have some mineralocorticoid activity. Aldosterone is secreted by the zona glomerulosa under the control of the renin–angiotensin system.

3. The sex steroids (predominantly androgens) are secreted in small amounts under normal conditions. The principal androgens are dehydroepiandrosterone, androstenedione and testosterone. Small quantities of oestrogens and progestogens are also secreted. Excess production may, however, cause significant clinical problems.

Clinical features of adrenocortical disease

Cushing's syndrome

Cushing's syndrome refers to the clinical disorders resulting from an excess of circulating glucocorticoid. The term 'Cushing's disease' is used to describe patients in whom the syndrome results from an increase in pituitary ACTH production. This is the commonest cause of spontaneous Cushing's syndrome.

Table 6. Causes of Cushing's syndrome.

ACTH dependent	ACTH independent
Spontaneous	
Hypothalamic-pituitary dependent (Cushing's disease)	Adrenal adenoma
Ectopic ACTH syndrome	Adrenal carcinoma
Iatrogenic	
ACTH therapy	Glucocorticoid therapy

Cushing's disease accounts for approximately 60 per cent of spontaneously occurring cases of Cushing's syndrome, ectopic causes for 15 per cent, adenomata for 15 per cent and carcinoma for 10 per cent.

The common modes of presentation are obesity, hirsutism, hypertension and symptoms related to premature spinal osteoporosis. Depression and other psychiatric disturbances are common. The diagnosis is frequently suggested by the characteristic clinical features (**460**). The most striking facial features are rounding of the face, plethora, hirsutism, loss of scalp hair, acne and pigmentation (**461** and **462**). The facial appearance will generally revert to normal after treatment (**463** before, and **464** after treatment).

460

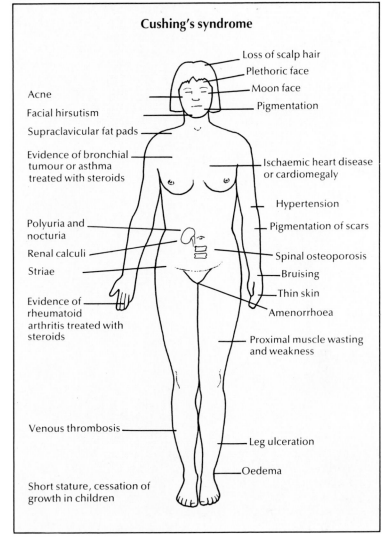

Cushing's syndrome

- Loss of scalp hair
- Plethoric face
- Moon face
- Pigmentation
- Acne
- Facial hirsutism
- Supraclavicular fat pads
- Evidence of bronchial tumour or asthma treated with steroids
- Ischaemic heart disease or cardiomegaly
- Hypertension
- Pigmentation of scars
- Polyuria and nocturia
- Renal calculi
- Striae
- Spinal osteoporosis
- Bruising
- Thin skin
- Amenorrhoea
- Evidence of rheumatoid arthritis treated with steroids
- Proximal muscle wasting and weakness
- Venous thrombosis
- Leg ulceration
- Oedema
- Short stature, cessation of growth in children

461

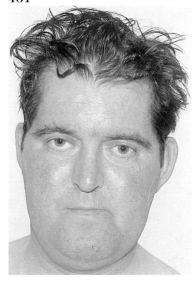

462

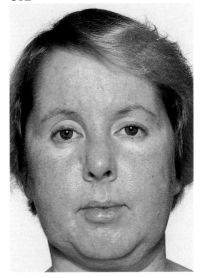

463

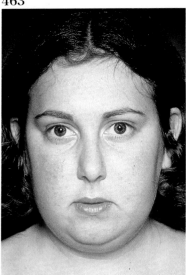

464

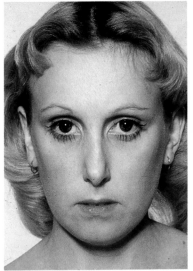

465

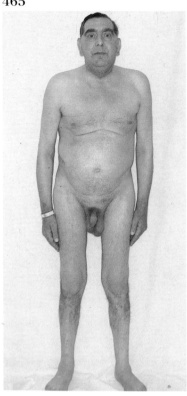

Metabolic changes. Major physical signs result from the metabolic changes. Increased fat deposition occurs in all fat depots. This is most evident in the face (moon face), the supraclavicular fossae, the region over
the lower cervical vertebrae (buffalo hump), the breasts and abdomen. The inappropriate slimness of the limbs can be attributed to muscle wasting (**465** to **467**).

466

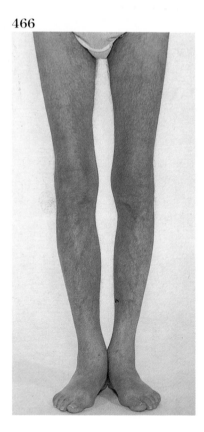

467

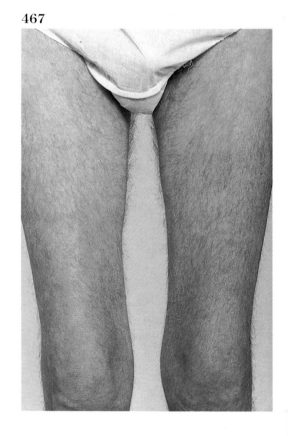

Muscle catabolism is increased leading to wasting and weakness (which may be increased by hypokalaemia). The weakness is generally most prominent in the proximal muscles; this can be demonstrated by observing the difficulty with which the patient rises from a crouching position without aid, as shown in this sequence of pictures (**468** to **476**).

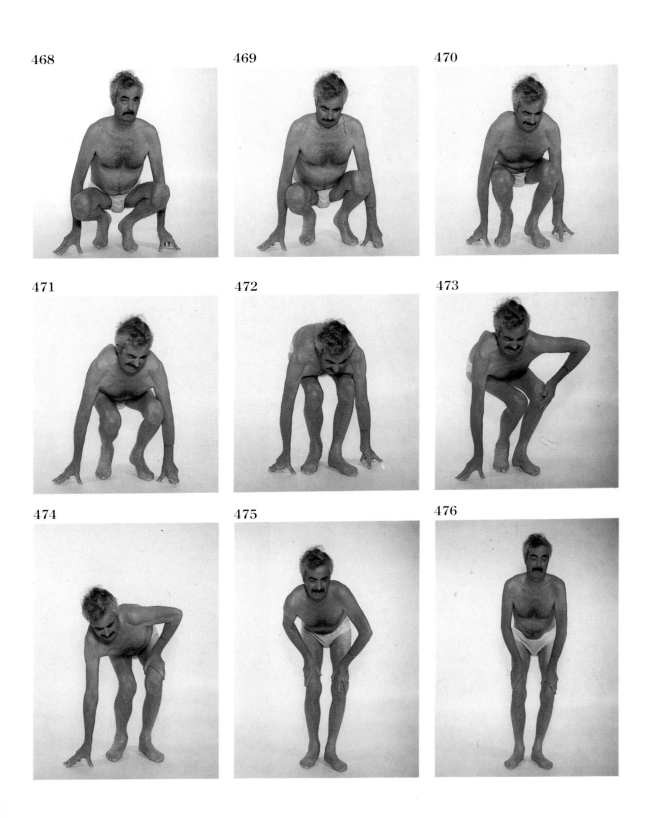

468

469

470

471

472

473

474

475

476

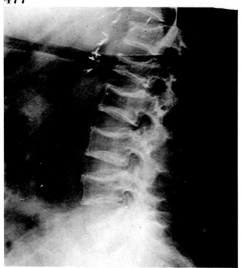

477

Increased protein catabolism may lead to osteoporosis with loss of height and pathological fractures (**477**). Characteristic thinning of the skin is caused by protein loss and leads to the formation of purple striae (**478** to **480**). Pale pink or white striae are seen in obesity, but they may also be purple in colour and differentiation on purely clinical grounds may be difficult.

478

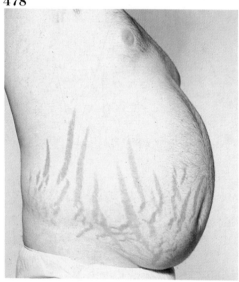

480

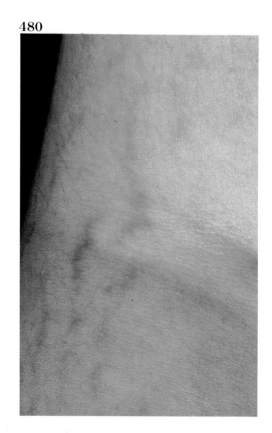

479

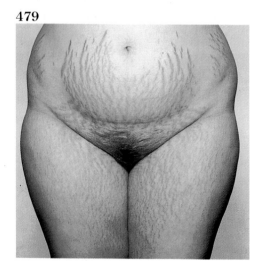

Skin thickness can be assessed by raising a skin fold on the back of the patient's hand (**481**) and comparing it with the skin on a normal hand (e.g. that of the examiner). The fragility of blood vessel walls is increased and there is loss of supporting subcutaneous tissues: these two factors lead to increased bruising (**482** and **483**). Local steroid application can cause similar skin changes and fragility of the tissues (**484**).

481

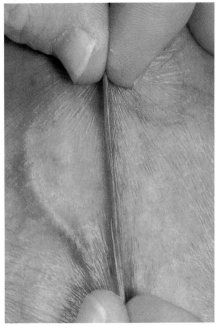

482

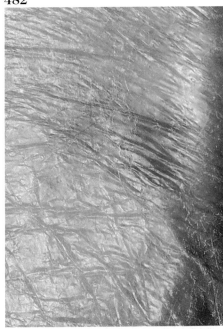

483

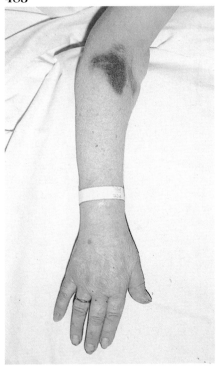

484

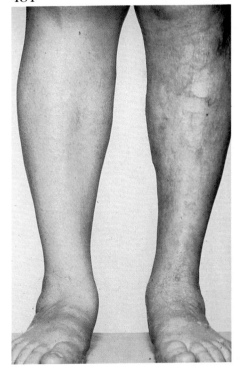

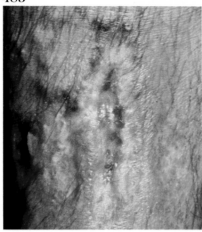

All tissues in Cushing's syndrome have a reduced tensile strength as a result of increased protein catabolism, and thus wound healing is poor and ulceration often results from minor trauma (**485**).

486

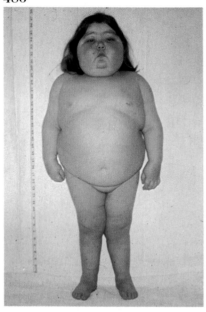

Growth retardation is seen in children and adolescents with Cushing's syndrome (**486**).

487

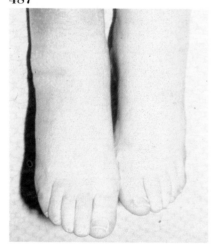

Excess glucocorticoids also lead to sodium retention, potassium loss and an increase in free water clearance. The sodium retention may lead to oedema (**487**) which contributes to the hypertension. Polyuria and nocturia are frequent symptoms. Cortisol has an anti-insulin action and also increases gluconeogenesis, and thus carbohydrate intolerance occurs in about half of patients with Cushing's disease (and in nearly all of those with the ectopic ACTH syndrome). Glycosuria, if present, will contribute to the polyuria.

Cardiovascular changes. Hypertension is common and there is an increased incidence of ischaemic heart disease (**488**), cerebrovascular disease and venous thrombosis (**489**). Heart failure and cardiac arrhythmias may occur in long-standing disease and the sodium retention and potassium loss resulting from the mineralo-corticoid effects of excess glucocorticoids contribute to these cardiovascular problems.

488

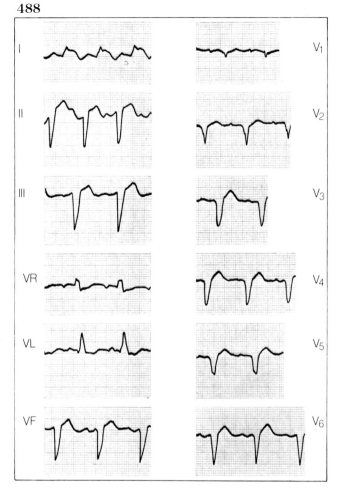

489

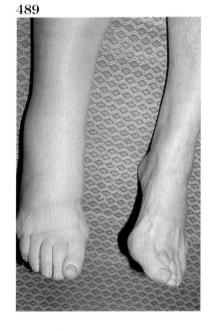

Psychiatric changes. These occur in about two-thirds of patients and include irritability, severe depression and major psychotic disturbances.

Abnormal androgen production. Usually only a minor increase in androgen production occurs in Cushing's disease. Amenorrhoea is almost invariable, hirsutism (**490** and **491**) and acne are common, but major degrees of virilisation are rare. **492** shows extensive male pattern baldness in a female with Cushing's disease.

490

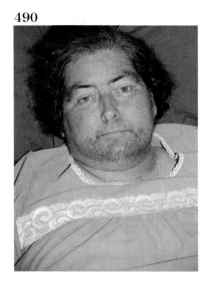

491

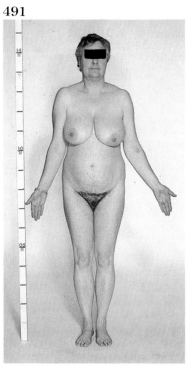

492

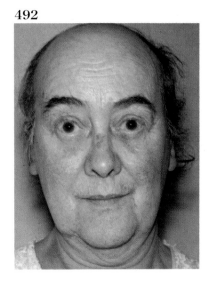

Increased ACTH production. ACTH is a pigmentary hormone and an increase in skin pigmentation is seen in some patients (**493**). The pigmentation is most marked in areas exposed to sunlight and friction and in scars (**494**). Pigmentation may become very marked after bilateral adrenalectomy for Cushing's disease. This form of treatment is followed by the post-adrenalectomy syndrome (Nelson's syndrome) in a proportion of patients (**495**). Expansion of the pituitary fossa and hyperpigmentation may be present and, rarely, cranial nerve palsies result from an expanding corticotroph adenoma.

493

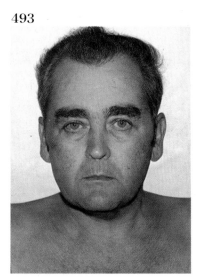

494

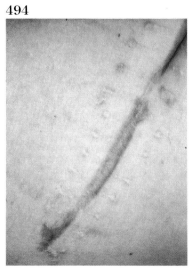

495

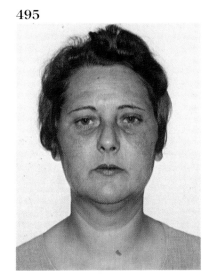

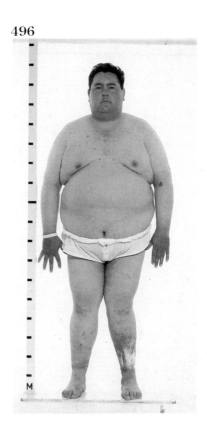

496

Diagnostic features. The investigation of Cushing's syndrome falls naturally into two parts: the confirmation of the diagnosis (i.e. the presence of hypercortisolism), and the identification of the cause. Many patients referred to endocrinologists are fat, hirsute or plethoric in appearance, or all three of these. The vast majority do not have Cushing's syndrome or any other identifiable endocrine disorder. **496** shows a patient with simple gross obesity and some clinical features of Cushing's syndrome. Patients with Cushing's syndrome must also be distinguished from those with pseudo-Cushing's syndrome caused by chronic alcoholism or depression. Depression may cause particular diagnostic problems as this is a common feature of Cushing's syndrome and patients with endogenous depression may not show a normal circadian rhythm of cortisol secretion. **497** shows an alcoholic with pseudo-Cushing's syndrome.

a) *Cushing's disease.* The diagnosis of Cushing's disease is confirmed by demonstrating hypercortisolism and a moderate elevation of ACTH.

497

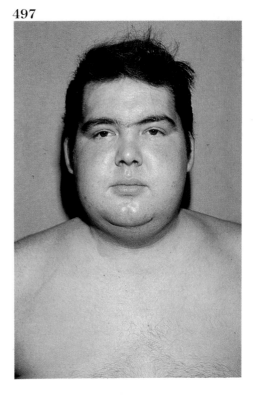

b) *Ectopic ACTH syndrome.* This form of Cushing's syndrome may result either from an overt malignant neoplasm, usually an oat cell carcinoma of the bronchus, or from an occult neoplasm, usually a carcinoid tumour. Overt ectopic ACTH syndrome follows a rapidly progressive clinical course. The typical facial appearance is not always apparent (**498**). The metabolic changes are frequently severe, reflecting the very high levels of ACTH and cortisol in this condition. Muscle weakness, wasting, weight loss, carbohydrate intolerance, hypokalaemia and oedema are particularly prominent features of this variety of ectopic ACTH syndrome.

Severe pigmentation is common because of the very high levels of ACTH (**499** and **500**). The ectopic ACTH syndrome is most commonly associated with bronchial carcinoma (**501** and **502**) and is, therefore, seen most frequently in males. It may, however, result from malignant tumours arising from a wide range of tissues. By contrast, the occult form of ectopic ACTH syndrome closely simulates Cushing's disease, with similar ACTH and cortisol levels. The causative neoplasm often does not become apparent for many years. Bronchial carcinoids are the most common cause (**503** and **504**).

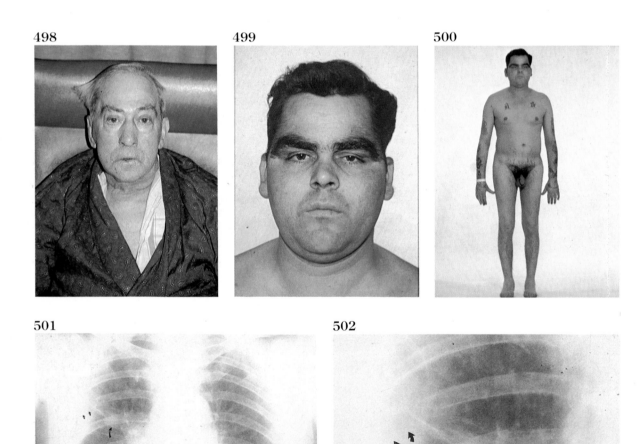

498

499

500

501

502

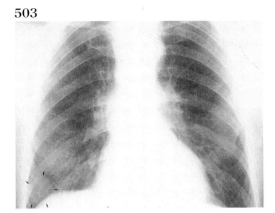

503

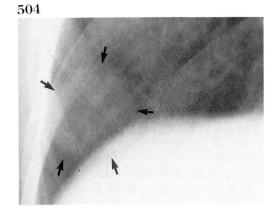

504

c) *Adrenal tumours.* Cushing's syndrome caused by an adrenal tumour frequently cannot be distinguished from Cushing's disease on clinical grounds. A major degree of androgen overproduction is seen in some patients, leading to marked virilisation (**505**). Rarely, the adrenal tumour may be palpable and liver enlargement may be seen. The tumour is usually identified by ultrasound or CT scan (**506** and **507**). **508**, **509** and **510** show a large left adrenal carcinoma causing renal distortion on IVP, and matching ultrasound and CT scans. Venography, angiography, labelled cholesterol scan or selective venous sampling have been used in the past but these have now been superseded by non-invasive techniques. The larger the tumour, the more likely it is to be malignant.

505

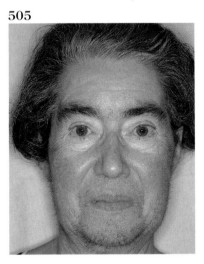

506

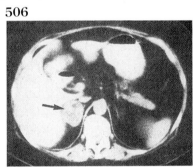

507

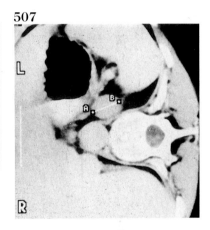

508

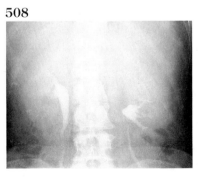

509

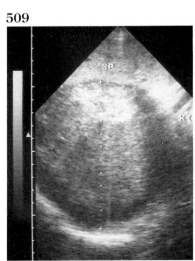

510

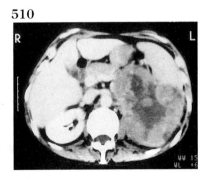

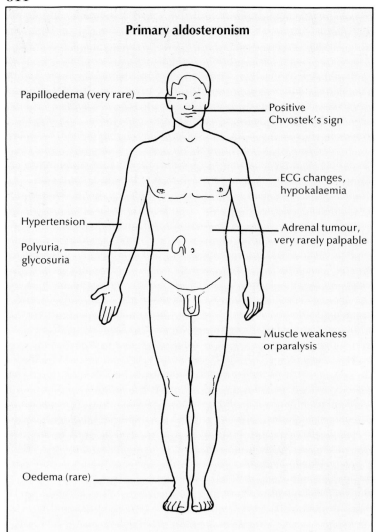

Primary aldosteronism

Papilloedema (very rare)

Positive Chvostek's sign

ECG changes, hypokalaemia

Hypertension

Adrenal tumour, very rarely palpable

Polyuria, glycosuria

Muscle weakness or paralysis

Oedema (rare)

Primary aldosteronism

Primary aldosteronism may result from an adrenal tumour (almost invariably an adenoma) or hyperplasia of the zona glomerulosa. The characteristic biochemical features are hyper-natraemia, hypokalaemia and suppression of renin production. Sodium retention leads to an increase in extra-cellular fluid volume (although oedema is rare) and, almost invariably, hypertension, although this is rarely malignant. Potassium loss leads to muscle weakness which may be sufficiently severe to cause periodic paralysis and impaired carbohydrate intolerance (**511**). Cardiac abnormalities are common and include ST-T depression, U waves and premature ventricular contractions (**512**). Hypokalaemia may lead to alkalosis (giving rise to tetany) and renal damage (leading to polyuria and secondary polydipsia). The tumour is usually small, but may be demonstrated by iodocholesterol scan, CT scan, aortography (**513**), venography or selective venous sampling. Less commonly primary aldosteronism may be caused by bilateral hyperplasia of the zona glomerulosa. Pathologically, the tumour has a characteristic yellow colour (**514** and **515**). **516** shows a scan of bilateral hyperplasia (the spleen and liver are indicated).

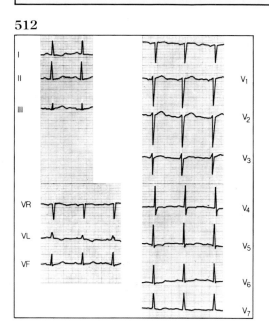

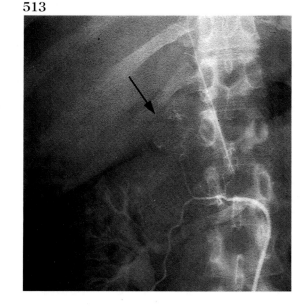

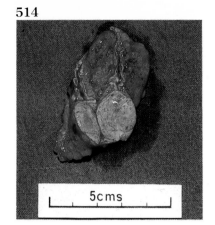

5cms

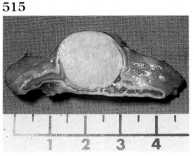

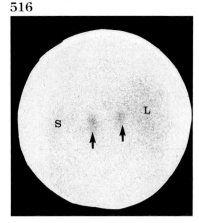

Hypoadrenalism

Chronic primary adrenocortical failure (Addison's disease) is usually caused by an autoimmune process (idiopathic Addison's disease) or more rarely by destruction of the glands by tuberculosis, other granulomatous disorders, or infiltration by metastases. Acute failure most commonly results from withdrawal of suppressive doses of steroids, surgical removal of the glands, or stress in patients with chronic failure. It may occasionally be precipitated by haemorrhage into the glands (Waterhouse–Friderichsen syndrome or anticoagulant therapy). The main clinical features are shown in **517**. These can be clearly related to the biochemical and pathological features of this disorder. (The features of adrenal deficiency secondary to hypothalamic-pituitary disease are described on page 16.)

Glucocorticoid deficiency. The major clinical manifestations are tiredness, weight loss, gastrointestinal disturbances, hypoglycaemia and depression (**518**).

517

Hypoadrenalism

- Drowsiness, confusion, coma
- Papilloedema
- Buccal pigmentation
- Goitre (Schmidt's syndrome)
- Skin pigmentation
- Evidence of asthma treated with steroids
- Tachycardia
- Reduced heart size
- Hypotension with postural drop
- Scars of previous adrenalectomy
- Anorexia, nausea and vomiting
- Hypothyroidism associated
- Pigmented scars
- Vitiligo
- Diarrhoea
- Loss of pubic hair in women
- Muscle weakness may be profound

518

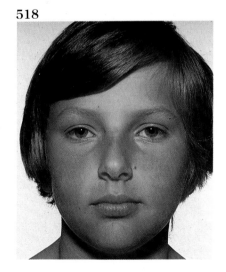

Mineralocorticoid deficiency. Dehydration and cramps are common. Reduced skin turgor (**519**) is evident in many patients. Hypotension, a low voltage ECG (**520**) and a reduced cardiac shadow on the chest radiograph (**521**) are common. These changes are all reversed by treatment (**522** ECG, and **523** radiograph of the same patient as shown in **520** and **521** after replacement treatment).

519

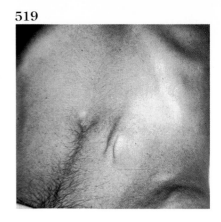

521

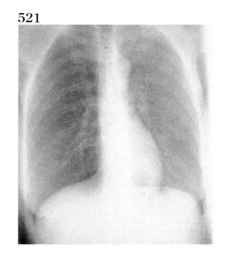

520

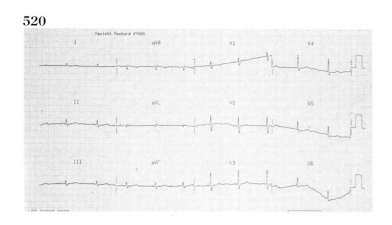

522

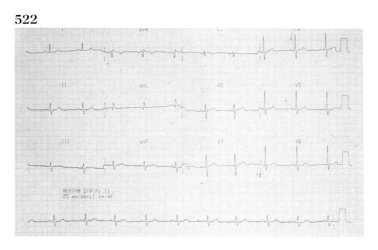

523

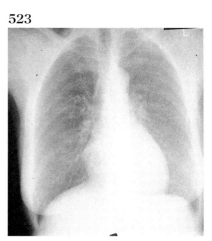

Androgen deficiency. This may lead to hair loss in the female from the scalp (**524**), axillary (**525**) and pubic regions (**526**).

524

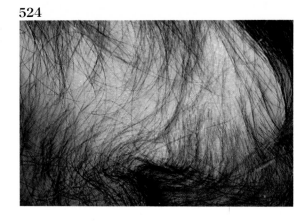

525

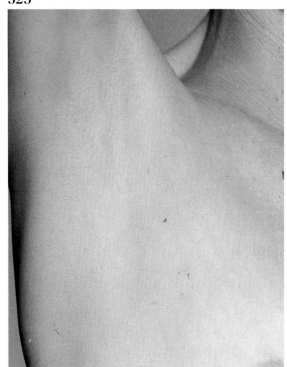

526

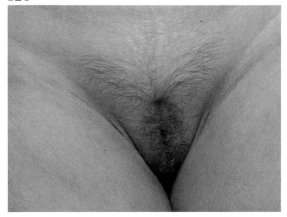

Excess ACTH production. The excess of ACTH production leads to excess pigmentation (as in Cushing's disease and Nelson's syndrome). **527** shows a patient with Addison's disease (on the right) photographed with her healthy twin sister.

527

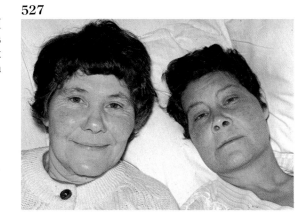

The pigmentation in excess ACTH production is generally most marked in exposed areas, skin creases and at areas of friction. **528** and **529** show pigmentation in the hands of patients (contrasted with a normal hand in **529**), **530** on the elbow, **531** in an area of friction from a brassière strap, and **532** to **534** on the buccal mucosa and gums.

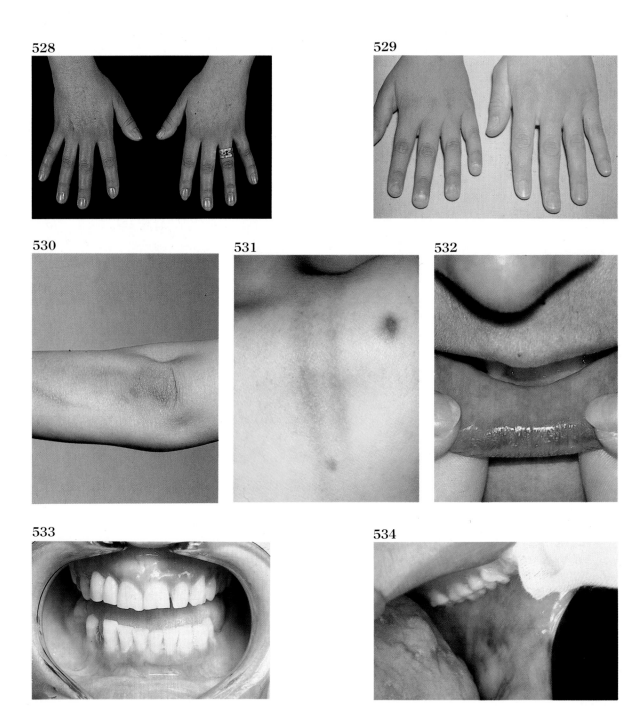

528

529

530

531

532

533

534

The pigmentation diminishes, with adequate ACTH suppression therapy (**535** before, and **536** after treatment). The pigmentation of melanosis (**537**), chloasma (**538**) or of racial origin may occasionally be confused with the pigmentation of hypoadrenalism.

535

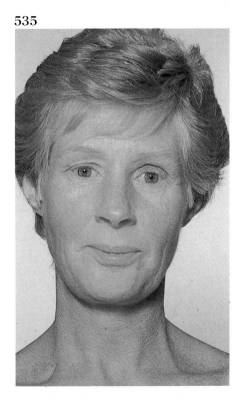

536

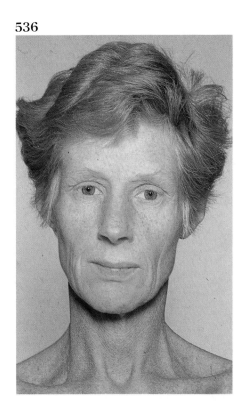

537

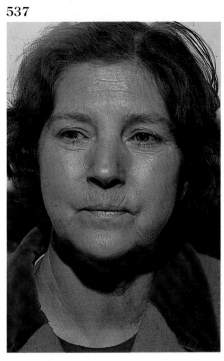

538

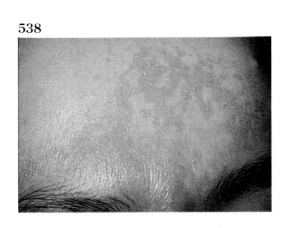

539

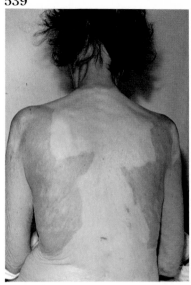

Associated features. Vitiligo (a skin marker of organ-specific autoimmune disease) may be seen and provides a striking contrast to the hyperpigmentation seen in other areas (**539**). There is an association with other organ-specific autoimmune disorders (autoimmune thyroid disease, primary hypoparathyroidism, pernicious anaemia and premature ovarian failure). Papilloedema is a rare complication (**540**) and resolves after treatment (**541**). Bilateral adrenal calcification may be seen in Addison's disease resulting from destruction of the glands by tuberculosis (**542**).

540

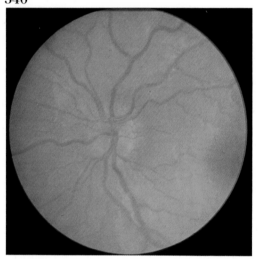

541

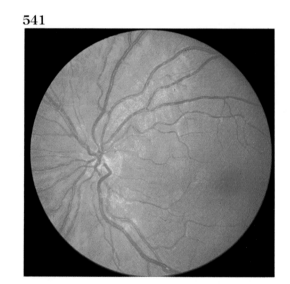

542

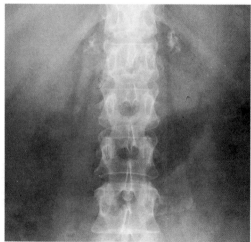

Congenital adrenal hyperplasia

The synthesis of the adrenal steroids is dependent upon a number of enzymatically regulated stages. Congenital deficiency of any of these stages results in the underproduction of some adrenal steroids and overproduction of others as biosynthesis is diverted down alternative metabolic pathways. Six identifiable varieties of congenital adrenal hyperplasia exist, each attributable to a specific enzyme deficiency:

1. 20-hydroxylase (cholesterol desmolase) deficiency
2. 3 ß-hydroxysteroid dehydrogenase deficiency
3. 17-hydroxylase deficiency
4. 21-hydroxylase deficiency
5. 11 ß-hydroxylase deficiency
6. 18-hydroxysteroid dehydrogenase deficiency

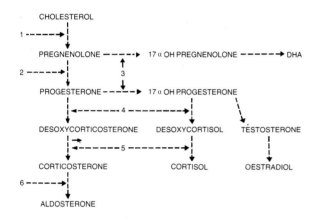

20-hydroxylase and 3ß-hydroxysteroid dehydrogenase deficiency. Patients with these disorders manifest severe glucocorticoid and mineralocorticoid deficiency from birth and require urgent replacement therapy. Problems of sexual differentiation occur as the infants are phenotypically female whether the genotype is XX or XY (see page 155). Delayed puberty presents problems in treated patients at a later age.

17-hydroxylase deficiency. This condition is characterised by hypertension caused by excessive production of desoxycorticosterone and corticosterone. Deficient androgen production may lead to problems of sexual differentiation or delayed puberty as in patients with 20-hydroxylase or 3 ß-hydroxysteroid deficiency.

21-hydroxylase deficiency. This is the commonest variety of congenital adrenal hyperplasia and is associated with pseudoprecocious puberty in the male and virilisation in the female. There are no phenotypic changes in the male at birth, but in the female varying degrees of masculinisation of the external and internal genitalia may lead to problems in the assignment of sex. In the salt-losing variety, which can effect either sex, mineralocorticoid deficiency may be severe and lead to hypotension and hyperkalaemia.

11ß-hydroxylase deficiency. This deficiency is characterised by pseudoprecocious puberty in the male and virilisation in the female, usually in association with hypertension (secondary to overproduction of desoxycorticosterone)

18-hydroxysteroid dehydrogenase deficiency. Deficiency of this enzyme leads to pure aldosterone deficiency causing hyperkalaemia, hyponatraemia and hypotension.

These conditions are considered in greater detail in the chapter on disorders of sexual development and differentiation (see pages 147 to 149 and 155 to 156).

Adrenal medulla

The catecholamines are important neurotransmitters and are secreted by tissues of neural crest origin. The major amines are dopamine, noradrenaline (norepinephrine) and adrenaline (epinephrine). The adrenal medullae are relatively minor sources of catecholamines. They are released under the influence of a variety of emotional, physical and pharmacological stimuli.

Phaeochromocytoma

Phaeochromocytoma is usually a pathologically benign tumour secreting catecholamines. Its importance lies in the potentially fatal effects of uncontrolled release of the catecholamines. Approximately 90 per cent of tumours are found in the adrenal medullae, the remainder being associated with other sympathetic tissue. The tumours may be multiple. It is generally said that about 10 per cent of tumours are bilateral, 10 per cent extramedullary, 10 per cent are malignant and 10 per cent occur in children. Very rarely similar clinical features may result from adrenomedullary hyperplasia. The characteristic clinical features result from the release of catecholamines into the circulation and are shown in **543**. The most important of these are the cardiovascular effects — intermittent or sustained hypertension, which is often very severe, tachycardia and palpitations. These may occur in paroxysmal attacks in association with blanching and sweating. Tremulousness, anxiety and disturbance of sleep are common additional manifestations. The first clinical manifestation of phaeochromocytoma may be a major cardiovascular complication of the severe hypertension — myocardial infarction, stroke, a major dysrhythmia or left ventricular failure. Phaeochromocytoma is a rare cause of hypertension, accounting for between one and five per thousand of all new cases of hypertension.

The diagnosis can usually be confirmed by assay of blood or urinary catecholamines or their metabolites. It may be necessary to collect samples on a number of occasions because of the paroxysmal nature of catecholamine secretion. Provocation tests using a number of agents have been used in the past but are not generally recommended as they may precipitate a dangerous hypertensive crisis. Phentolamine will lower the blood pressure in most patients with phaeochromocytoma, but will do so also in a number of individuals with essential hypertension.

543

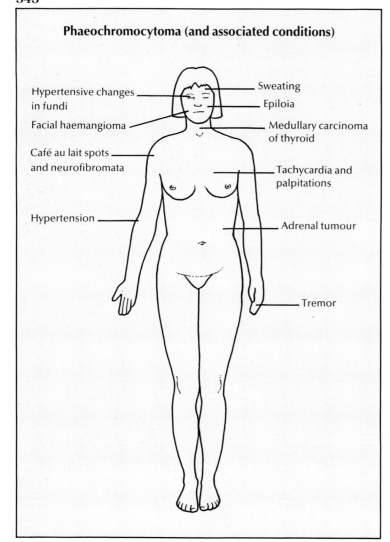

Phaeochromocytoma (and associated conditions)

Hypertensive changes in fundi

Facial haemangioma

Café au lait spots and neurofibromata

Hypertension

Sweating

Epiloia

Medullary carcinoma of thyroid

Tachycardia and palpitations

Adrenal tumour

Tremor

Phaeochromocytomas can usually be localised by CT scan (**544**) or ultrasound (**545**). Occasionally calcification can be seen on x-ray. Radioisotope scanning can be carried out with mIBG (metaiodobenzylguanidine) which is taken up by chromaffin tissue. **546** shows a benign phaeochromocytoma with renal outlines indicated, and **547** shows metastases from a malignant phaeochromocytoma in the skull. **548** shows a malignant phaeochromocytoma. The upper red image is a computed tomography image showing a solitary tumour, and the upper green image is a single photon emission tomography image of functioning tumour mass with ^{123}I mIBG. The lower image shows superimposition of anatomical and functional images.

544

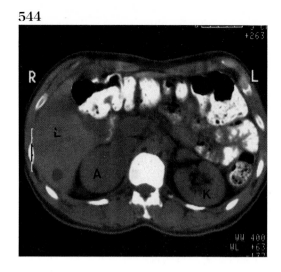

545

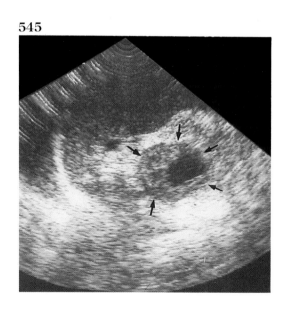

546

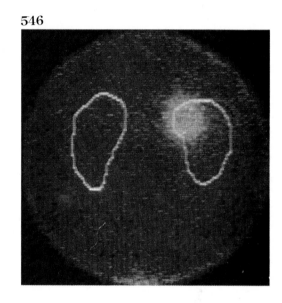

547

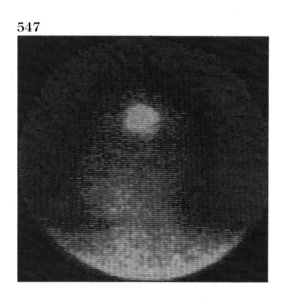

548

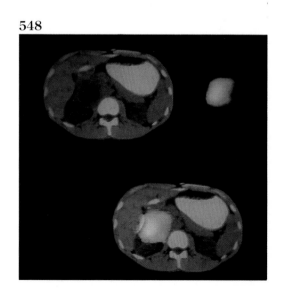

549

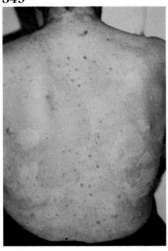

There is an association between phaeochromocytoma and the neuro-ectodermal diseases, most frequently with neurofibromatosis (**549** to **551**). An association with von Hippel–Lindau's disease (neural haemangiomas, visceral cysts and hypernephroma) is also seen (**552**).

550

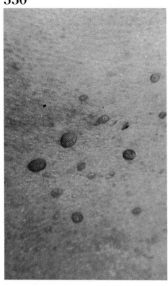

551

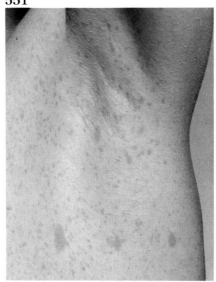

552

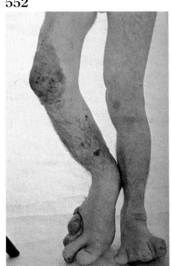

Phaeochromocytoma may also occur in Sturge–Weber disease — encephalo-facial angiomatosis (**553** shows the facial appearance, **554** to **556** show the typical gyral calcification, and **557** associated adenoma sebaceum).

Phaeochromocytoma also occurs in association with the familial form of medullary carcinoma of the thyroid — Sipple's syndrome (**558**).

553

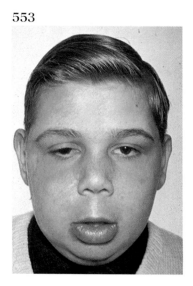

554

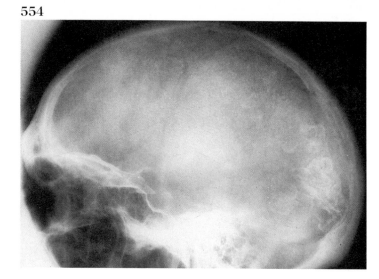

555

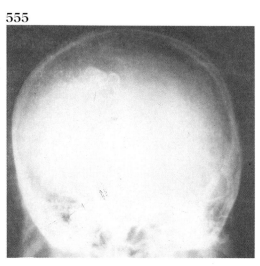

556

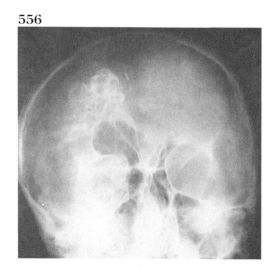

557

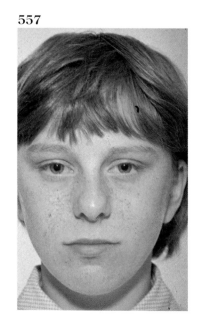

558

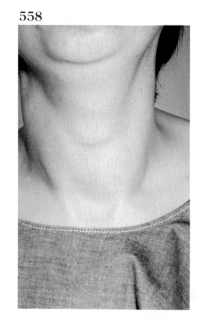

Chapter 5
Disorders of sexual development, differentiation and reproductive function

Introduction

It is commonly assumed that the distinction between male and female is absolute. Normal sexual development is controlled by a number of factors and gender may be determined by investigating these differentiating factors. Thus sexual identity is established by observing the following:

- Chromosomal sex
- Gonadal sex
- Genital sex
- Hormonal sex
- Psychological sex

Normal subjects show concordance between these characteristics; problems occur if there is discordance. The appearance of the external genitalia is normally used to identify the sex of a neonate; thus the clinical problems of sexual development and differentiation will be classified as to whether they are seen in the phenotypic male, the phenotypic female or in intermediate clinical states.

Disorders in phenotypic males

Chromosomal disorders

Klinefelter's syndrome

This syndrome is a chromosomally determined disorder in which there is seminiferous tubule dysgenesis. The testes are very small and firm and this may be the only abnormality detectable before puberty. Adult patients are generally tall (**559**) and may have gynecomastia (**560**). There is an increased risk of carcinoma of the breast (**561**). The testes remain very small (**562**) and, although secondary sexual characteristics develop at puberty, pubic and body hair tends to be sparse and the penis tends to be small. Patients are invariably sterile and potency may be reduced. Fine wrinkling of the skin reflects the hypogonadal state later in life (**563** and **564**). These patients have an XXY chromosome constitution (**565**) and are chromatin positive. The diagnosis can also be made in utero by culturing cells from the amniotic fluid. **566** shows a fetus with Klinefelter's syndrome, terminated after prenatal diagnosis, with normal male appearance at a relatively early stage of development. Other sex chromosome abnormalities associated with the Klinefelter phenotype include 46,XY/47,XXY mosaicism, 48,XXYY, 48,XXXY, 49,XXXXY and 49,XXXYY. These abnormalities are usually associated with mental retardation.

559

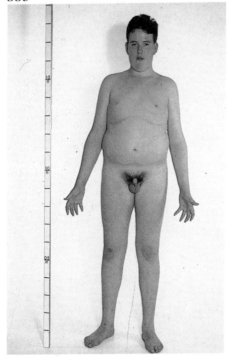

560

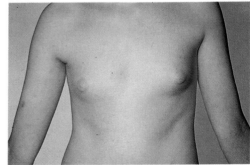

561

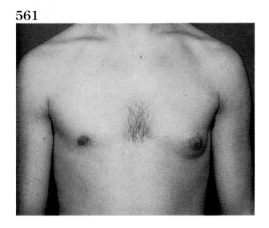

562

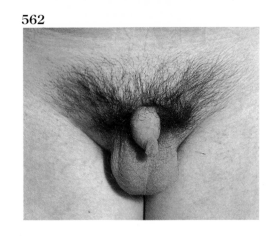

563

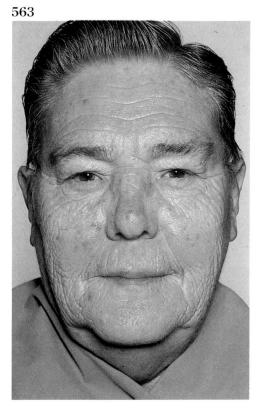

564

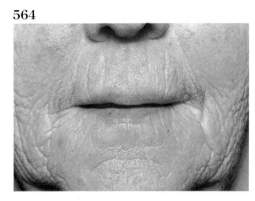

565

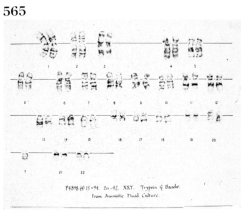

566

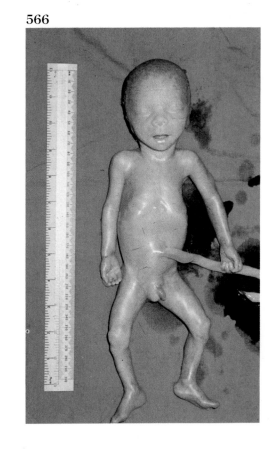

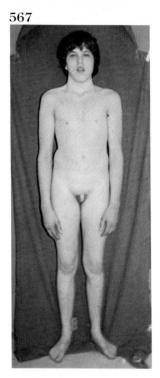

567

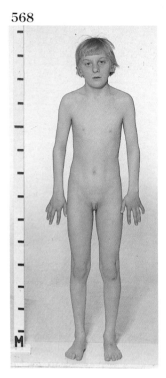

568

Ullrich–Turner syndrome ('male' Turner's syndrome, pseudo-Turner's syndrome, Noonan's syndrome).

The characteristics of this syndrome, which occurs in males with a normal XY karyotype, are shortness of stature with the somatic characteristics of Turner's syndrome (**567** and **568**, see also pages 150 to 153). The external genitalia are usually normal, although cryptorchidism may be present and the testes are small or impalpable (**569**). Puberty does not develop. Webbing of the neck is common (**570**), the ears may be low-set and abnormal (**571** and **572**), hypertelorism may be present and ocular anomalies (particularly ptosis) may be seen. Other abnormalities include shortening of one or more of the metacarpals (**573**), mental retardation, congenital heart disease and gynaecomastia. Pectus excavatum may also be present (**574**).

569

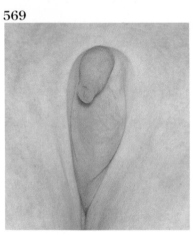

570

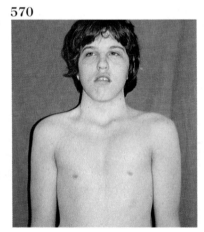

571

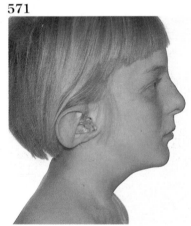

572

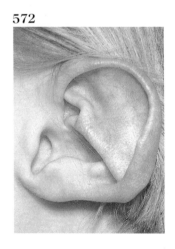

573

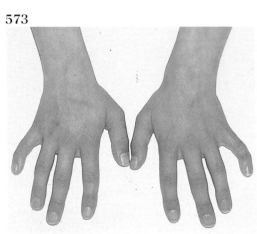

574

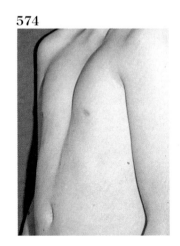

XX male

Male patients with an XX karyotype exhibit sex reversal. The testes are small and firm and histologically resemble those seen in Klinefelter's syndrome. The external genitalia are small and gynaecomastia may also be present (**575** and **576**).

575

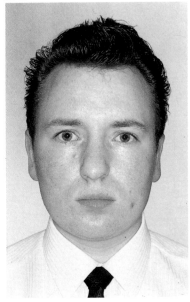

576

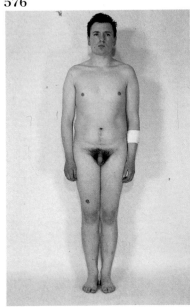

XXXXY disorder

Patients with this chromosomal disorder are invariably mentally retarded, have cryptorchidism and exhibit a number of skeletal disorders (particularly radio-ulnar dysostosis or overgrowth of radial and ulnar heads). Three Barr bodies are seen on the buccal smear (**577**).

577

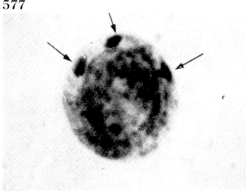

XXXY disorder

These patients have a syndrome similar to that seen in the XXXXY disorder and Klinefelter's syndrome. Mental retardation and skeletal abnormalities are common, but the testes are similar in size to those seen in Klinefelter's syndrome. Two Barr bodies are seen on the buccal smear (**578**).

578

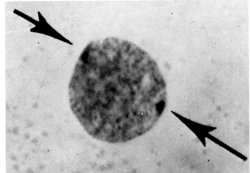

XYY disorder (579)

Patients with this disorder tend to be tall, have varicosities of the superficial veins and occasionally are hypogonadal. Their behaviour is sometimes aggressive and antisocial (580).

579

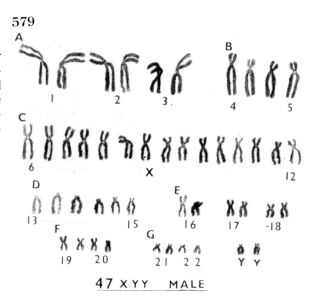

47 XYY MALE

580

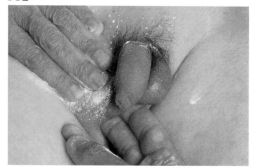

Cryptorchidism

Undescended testes are common at birth (occurring in about 10 per cent of all male births) but normal descent will take place in most patients. The testes remain in the abdomen or inguinal canal in true cryptorchidism and the scrotal sac is empty (581). A high proportion show abnormalities of development, and there is a risk of malignancy. True cryptorchidism must be distinguished from the much commoner 'pseudo-cryptorchidism' or retractile testes which can be massaged into the scrotum (582). Reduced fertility and impaired development of secondary sexual characteristics are common in cryptorchidism.

581

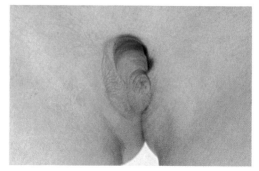

582

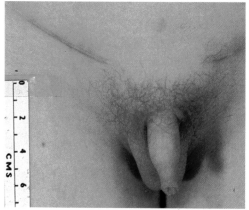

Testicular agenesis (anorchia)

Patients with testicular agenesis commonly have a male phenotype; thus testicular failure must have occurred after the seventh to fourteenth week of fetal life, because failure before this age will give rise to a female phenotype. The patients generally have small palpable masses in the scrotum, the vas deferens is palpable and development is normal until the age of puberty. The condition may be familial. The small flat scrotal sac is shown in **583** (some pubic hair is present because the patient was given a small dose of exogenous androgen). Note the scars of the previous operation to exclude undescended testes.

583

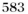

Reifenstein's syndrome

This syndrome is the association of hypospadias and post-pubertal testicular atrophy affecting both spermatogenesis and endocrine function. The scrotum is bifid (**584** and **585**). Eunuchoidism and gynaecomastia complete the clinical picture. The syndrome is limited to males and is inherited either as an X-linked recessive or a male limited autosomal dominant.

584

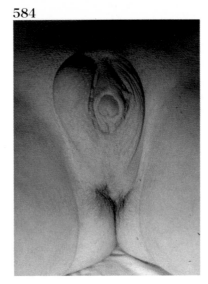

585

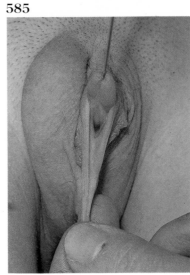

Congenital adrenal hyperplasia

21-hydroxylase deficiency

The severity of the abnormalities varies considerably. The female presents at birth with ambiguous genitalia with clitoral hypertrophy and partial or complete fusion of the labioscrotal folds (**586** and **587**). The patients are often mistaken for males with cryptorchidism and hypospadias.

586

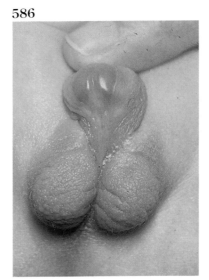

587

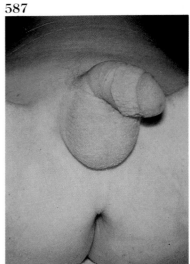

588

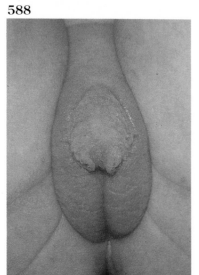

589

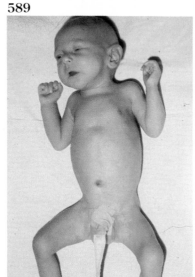

In milder forms of 21-hydroxylase deficiency clitoral hypertrophy may be minor (**588**), and in these cases patients will be correctly identified as female. The condition is generally unrecognised in the male unless it is very severe and associated with salt-wasting and hypotension (**589**). The condition may be mimicked by maternal ingestion of progestogens (**590**). Pigmentation of the nipples may result from high ACTH levels (**591**). Suppression therapy with corticosteroids is difficult and often unsatisfactory, leading to iatrogenic Cushing's syndrome (**592**) and advanced bone age — **593** shows a child of 4 years with a bone age of 9.6 years. **594** to **596** show siblings with 21-hydroxylase deficiency who were inadequately treated leading to shortness, and in the female a degree of masculinisation.

590

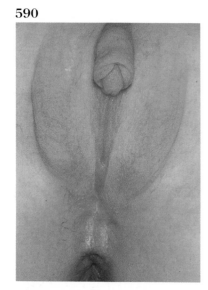

591

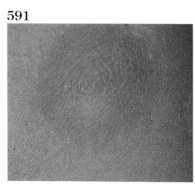

592

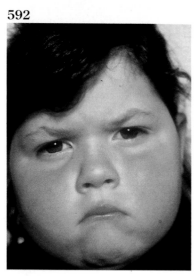

593

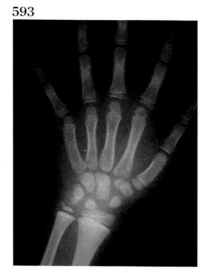

594

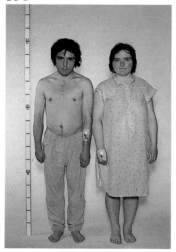

595

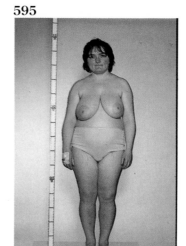

596

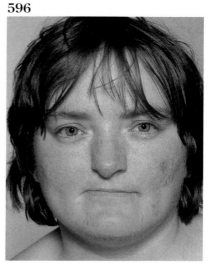

597

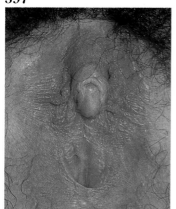

598

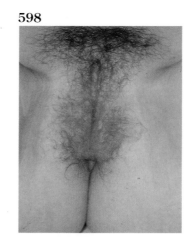

Corrective surgery to the genitalia is helpful, and **597** and **598** show the appearance before and after the operation. Reassignment of sex is worthwhile if the diagnosis is overlooked. **599** and **600** show a 16-year-old girl before and after treatment.

599

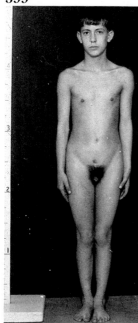

600

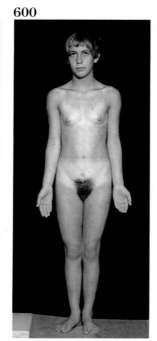

11 ß-hydroxylase deficiency

The clinical features of this syndrome resemble those of 21-hydroxylase deficiency with respect to sexual development (**601**), but clinically 11 ß-hydroxylase deficiency can usually be distinguished by the presence of hypertension. It is much less common than 21-hydroxylase deficiency.

601

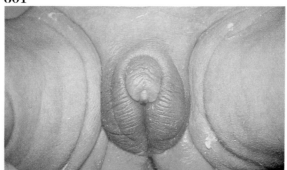

Disorders in phenotypic females

Chromosomal disorders

Turner's syndrome

The only important chromosome disorder in phenotypic females is Turner's syndrome, which occurs in about 1 in 10,000 live female births, and its variants. This is a chromosomally determined disorder where complete ovarian agenesis is present with deletion of one X chromosome (karyotype 45,XO). Incomplete forms may be seen with mosaicism (XO/XX, XO/XXX, XO/XX/XXX), in which case the patient may be chromatin positive. The condition can be diagnosed in utero by ultrasound and by chromosomal analysis. The neonate with Turner's syndrome may show lymphoedema (**602**) a low hair line, redundant skin at the base of the neck (**603**) and dysmorphic features (**604**). Turner's syndrome is generally suspected on clinical grounds by the association of primary amenorrhoea, sexual immaturity, shortness of stature (**605**) and the characteristic stigmata which include webbing of the neck (affecting about 40 per cent of patients) and increased carrying angle at the elbow (cubitus valgus, **606**). The chest tends to be square and the nipples are small and widely spaced (**607**). Examination of the face may reveal epicanthal folds, micrognathia, a fish-like mouth, deformed or low-set ears (**608**) and/or a low hair line. The fingers are short and stubby (**609**) and the hands may show puffiness of the dorsum and a short fourth metacarpal **610**, which is demonstrated clinically by asking the patient to make a fist (**611**).

Other anomalies which may be seen include lymphoedema of the feet and hands, an excess of pigmented naevi and a tendency to keloid formation.

602

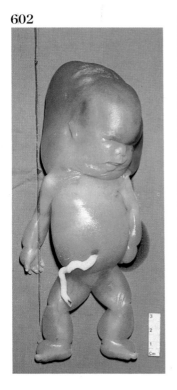

603

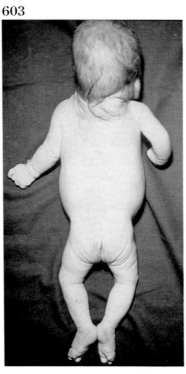

604

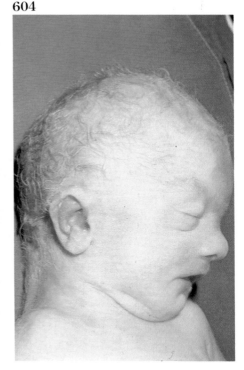

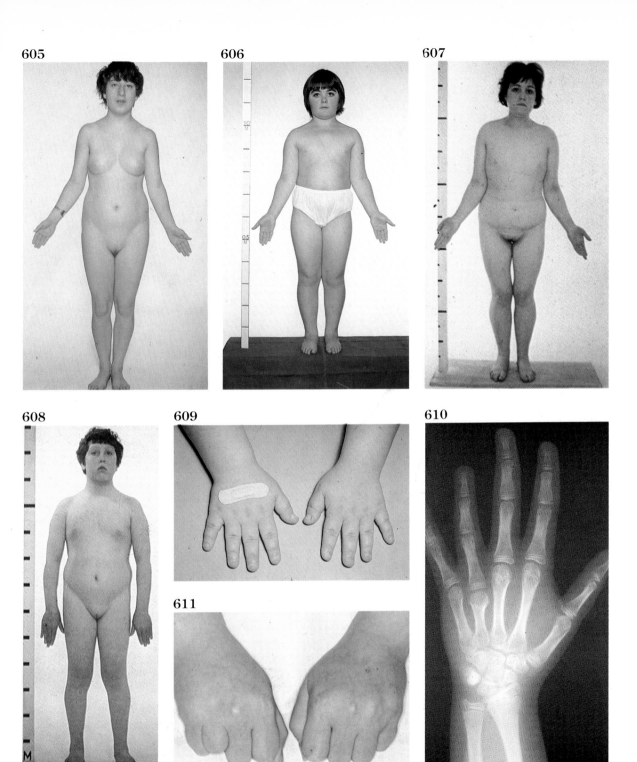

605

606

607

608

609

611

610

612

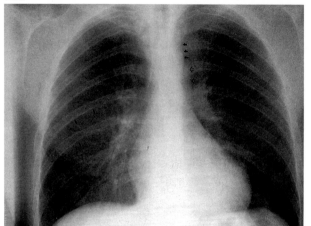

613

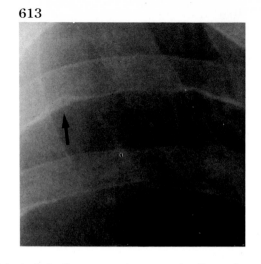

614

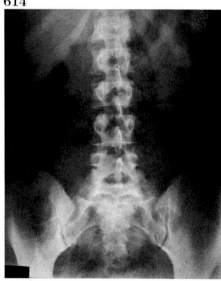

A number of radiological findings may be seen in Turner's syndrome, including effusions into serous cavities and the features of coarctation of the aorta (**612** shows an abnormal aortic contour — curved arrows; and rib-notching — straight arrows, also shown in **613**). Pyelography may reveal a horseshoe kidney or anomalies of the renal pelvis or ureters (**614** shows renal agenesis of the right kidney). Skeletal anomalies include rounding of the medial femoral condyle and squaring of the lateral condyle with a bony spur. Turner's syndrome may be associated with autoimmune disorders such as hypothyroidism, diabetes mellitus, leuchotrichia (**615**), vitiligo (**616**) and halo naevi (**617**). The diagnosis can be confirmed by the typical 45,XO chromosome picture (**618**) and the absence of Barr bodies (**619**). A variety of other karyotypes can be associated with the Turner's phenotype. These include 45,Xi(Xq) with one normal X and one with an isochromosome for the long arms (**620**), and rare karyotypes such as 46,X,del(Xq) or 46, (XXq−) where distal portions of the long arms of one of the X chromosomes have been lost or deleted (**621**). Most such patients have primary amenorrhoea but some do menstruate, suggesting that normal gonadal development can take place when at least some of the Xq genes are present. The karyotypes 46,X,del(Xp) or 46,(XXp−) show deletion of the short arm of one of the X chromosomes (**622**). The clinical picture is similar to typical Turner's syndrome. Clitoral hypertrophy in childhood (**623**) and virilisation at puberty (**624**) are seen in Turner's mosaics with a Y cell line. These patients are at high risk for the development of gonadal tumours.

615

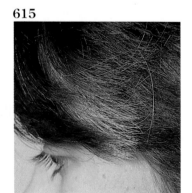

616

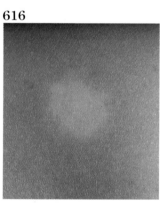

617

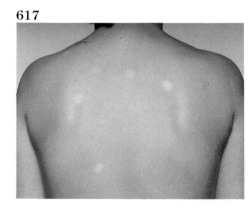

618

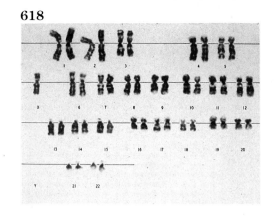

619

**Turner's
syndrome**

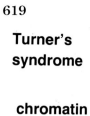

**chromatin
negative**

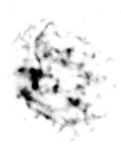

620

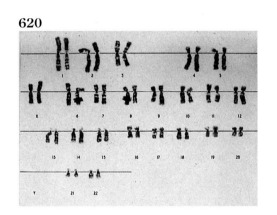

621

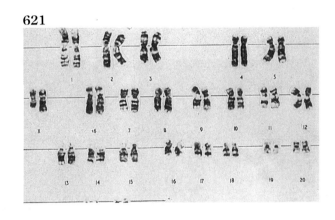

622

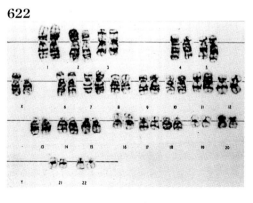

623

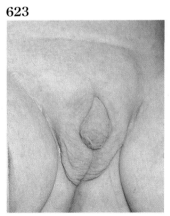

624

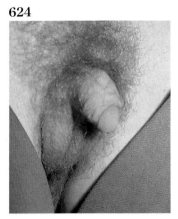

625

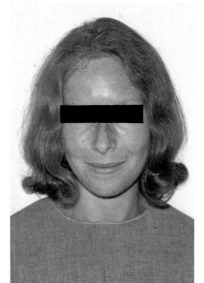

626

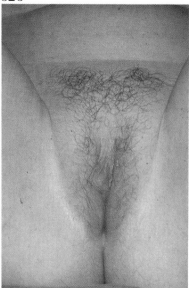

627

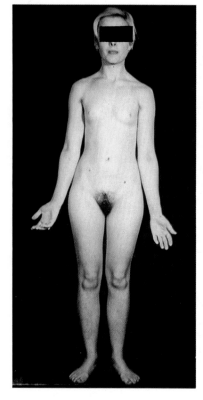

628

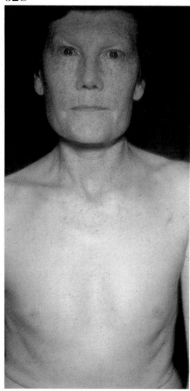

Gonadal dysgenesis

Pure gonadal dysgenesis may be associated with XX or XY karyotype and streak gonads. The patients are phenotypically female (**625**) and generally of normal or above average height. They present with sexual infantilism and primary amenorrhoea at the time of puberty. The genitalia remain immature in the absence of treatment (**626**). A eunuchoid body habitus is seen in XY gonadal dysgenesis (**627**). Incomplete forms may be seen and are associated with varying degrees of differentiation of the external genitalia and the gonads. A high risk of tumour formation is present in dysgenetic gonads, particularly in the XY form. Gonadal calcification may be seen on x-ray. Lack of oestrogens can predispose to early vascular disease (**628**, a patient with Turner's syndrome with premature coronary heart disease).

Mixed gonadal dysgenesis is generally associated with 45,XO/ 46,XY mosaicism. The external genitalia are female or ambiguous and virilisation tends to occur at the time of puberty. There is a high risk of tumour formation in the streak gonads, as in pure gonadal dysgenesis, and patients should undergo gonadectomy. Affected subjects should be reared as females.

Congenital adrenal hyperplasia

20–22 desmolase deficiency

Infants with this anomaly have female external genitalia (whether the karyotype is XX or XY). These infants suffer from severe salt-wasting and rarely survive.

3 ß-hydroxysteroid dehydrogenase deficiency

Most reported cases have died in infancy, but patients with partial defects survive causing male pseudo-hermaphroditism in the male and partial masculinisation in the female (**629**).

17-hydroxylase deficiency

This disorder is characterised by a failure to synthesise or secrete oestrogens or androgens. Sexual infantilism in a phenotypic female in association with hypertension is the characteristic finding in this group (**630**).

Abnormalities of androgen synthesis and action

5 α-reductase deficiency

5 α-reductase is the enzyme which converts testosterone to its more active form — dihydrotestosterone. Deficiency is associated with a very small penis, hypospadias, a bifid scrotum and a urogenital sinus which opens into a blind vaginal sac. Affected children are usually reared as females, although a substantial degree of virilisation occurs at puberty (**631**). The patients should normally be treated by clitorectomy, gonadectomy, vaginoplasty and oestrogen therapy at puberty. This disorder has been reported to occur with high frequency in males in the Dominican Republic where 'conversion' to male habitus and psychosexual orientation apparently occurs successfully at puberty. It would be unwise to assume that the same reorientation could be achieved successfully in other environments.

629

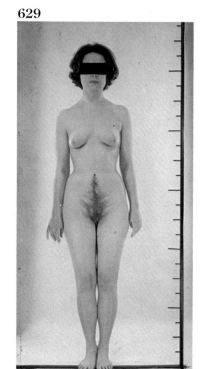

630

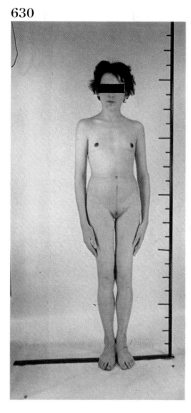

631

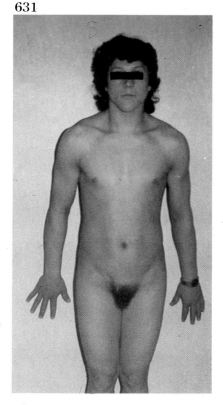

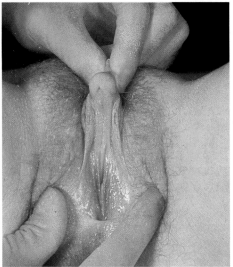

632

17-ketosteroid reductase deficiency

This a rare disorder associated with ambiguous genitalia (**632**).

Complete testicular feminisation

This is a highly distinctive inherited disorder in which half of the genotypic males in an affected family are phenotypically female. There is a tissue resistance to androgens and thus wolffian duct structures are poorly (though partially) developed. Complete involution of the müllerian ducts is present as 'müllerian inhibiting substance' is produced normally. The external genitalia are female. The 'vagina' is shallow and ends in a blind pouch. The testes are poorly developed and are found in the labia majora (**633** and **634**), inguinal canals or intra-abdominally. The Leydig cells become hyperplastic at the time of puberty and tend to form adenomata. Female secondary sexual characteristics develop during the second decade. Rounding of the body contours with generally well-developed breasts occurs. Feminisation probably results from increased oestrogen levels (for a male), which are driven by the relatively high gonadotrophins because of the insensitivity of the normal feedback mechanism to androgens. Sexual hair is scanty or absent (**635**). The patients should be reared as females and should undergo a gonadectomy as there is an increased risk of malignancy.

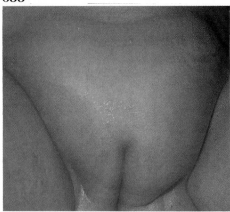

633

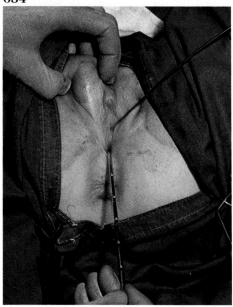

634

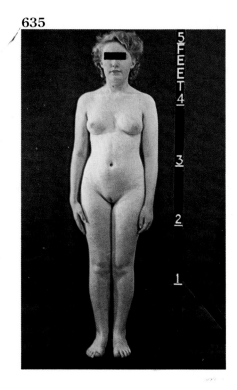

635

156

Incomplete testicular feminisation

This is a variant of the above syndrome in which there is some phallic enlargement and partial labioscrotal fusion (**636** and **637**). Breast development is less marked at puberty and hirsutism or partial virilisation may be evident (**638**).

636

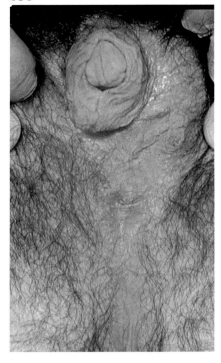

637

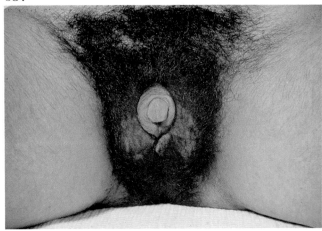

Absent or anomalous genitalia

Absence or anomalous development of the fallopian tubes, uterus and/or vagina may occur, and the latter may pose gender identification problems. These anomalies do not have an endocrine cause. They may be associated with congenital absence of one kidney (**639** shows a nephrogram on the left side only at aortography).

638

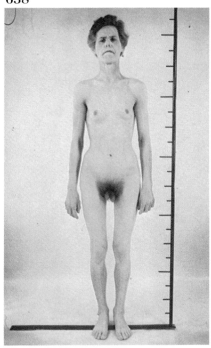

639

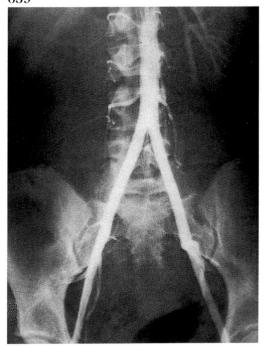

Intermediate phenotypes

Some of the conditions described above may have intermediate phenotypes, particularly chromosomal mosaics and some forms of congenital adrenal hyperplasia and disorders of testosterone biosynthesis.

Fragile X syndrome

This rare syndrome may be associated with a predominantly male or female phenotype. The fragile X chromosome can be demonstrated under specific culture conditions (**640**). It is associated with mental retardation (**641** and **642**) and with very large testes (**643**) in those with a male phenotype. (**641** is reproduced by permission of the *Journal of Mental Deficiency Research*, 1987; **31**: 81–85.)

640

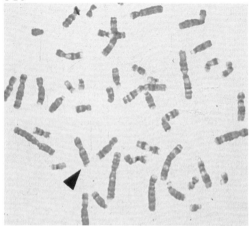

641

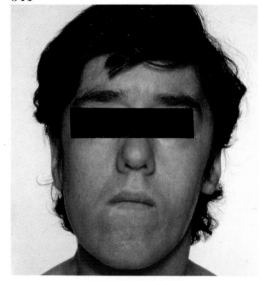

642

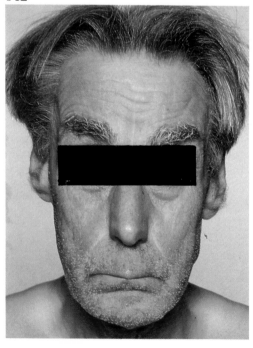

643

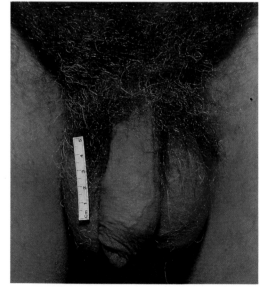

True hermaphroditism

True hermaphroditism is a rare condition and the diagnosis depends upon the finding of ovarian and testicular tissue in the same subject, in either the same or different gonads. The external genitalia are variable and predominantly male or female forms are seen, but the genitalia are ambiguous in most cases (**644**). Most patients, however, are reared as males because of the size of the phallus. Hypospadias is almost invariably present and there is a variable degree of fusion of the labioscrotal folds. The gonads may be located in the labioscrotal folds, the inguinal canal or the abdomen. The genital ducts are generally female in those patients with bilateral ovotestes, but in patients with an ovary on one side and a testis on the other the genital duct development generally follows the gonad on that side. Some breast development is present in about two-thirds of patients (**645**). Chromosomal examination reveals a 46,XX constitution in about 45 per cent of patients, 46,XY in about 20 per cent, and mosaics in the remainder.

644

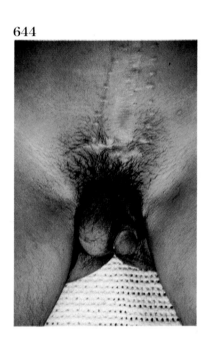

645

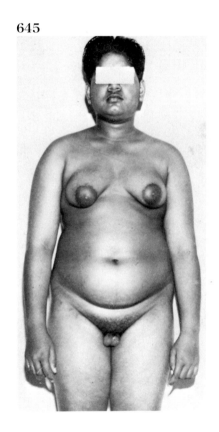

Errors of testosterone synthesis

Ambiguous genitalia may be seen in patients with deficiency of a number of enzymes — cholesterol desmolase, 3 ß-hydroxysteroid dehydrogenase, 17 α-hydroxylase, 17, 20-desmolase, or 17 ß-hydroxysteroid dehydrogenase. All these conditions are rare.

These abnormalities also affect the adrenal cortex (see also page 137). The first two are associated with salt-wasting and 17 α-hydroxylase deficiency wiith hypertension.

646

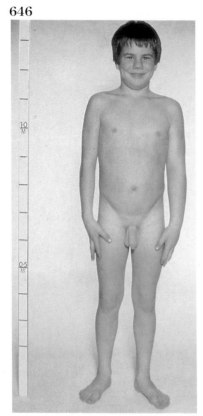

Disorders presenting as precocious puberty

Males

Precocious puberty in males is generally defined as the onset of pubertal changes before 10 years of age. This is an arbitrary but useful criterion.

647

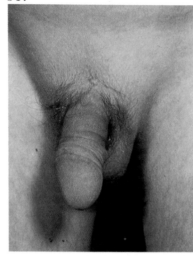

True precocious puberty

Forty per cent of males with pubertal development before 10 years of age have no detectable organic disease (**646**). The diagnosis can be made only by excluding other causes of precocious puberty. Familial examples have been described. **647** shows the genitalia of an 8-year-old boy with true precocious puberty.

648

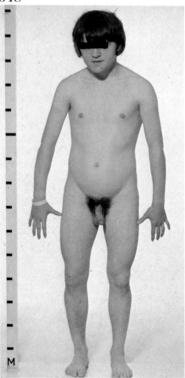

Congenital adrenal hyperplasia

21-hydroxylase and 11 ß-hydroxylase deficiencies (v.s.) may lead to precocious puberty. The onset of the pubertal changes occurs between 2 and 10 years of age, although testicular development does not occur and the patients are not fertile. There is a period of rapid growth, increased muscularity and the early appearance of pubic and axillary hair. Acne may be marked. The two conditions may be distinguished clinically by the occurrence of hypertension in 11 ß-hydroxylase deficiency. Premature epiphyseal fusion occurs and thus the adult height of the patients is reduced (**648**).

Miscellaneous causes

Precocious puberty may be associated with a number of cerebral tumours which affect the hypothalamus. The presence of hypothalamic disease may be suggested by changes in behaviour, sleep pattern or feeding habit. The presence of a glioma may be suggested by the finding of neurofibromatosis (see page 140). A rare but well-documented association exists between hypothyroidism and sexual precocity, which may result from an associated hypothalamic disturbance. Precocious puberty is occasionally seen in hepatoblastomas and in polyostotic fibrous dysplasia (Albright's syndrome) (**649** and **650** show the typical pigmentation limited by the midline, and **651** and **652** the prominence of an eye resulting from an underlying bone lesion).

649

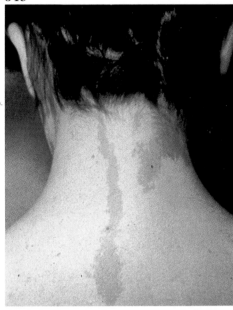

650

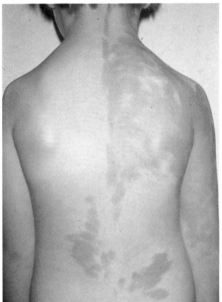

651

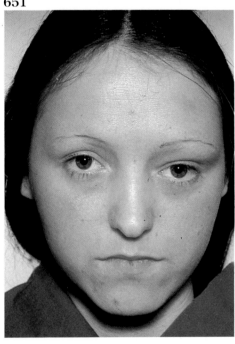

652

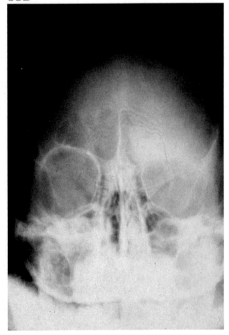

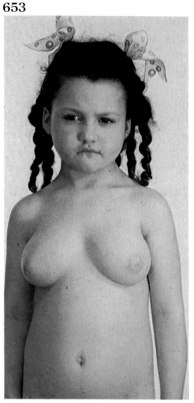

Females

Precocious puberty in females is generally defined as the onset of sexual maturation before the age of 8 years.

True precocious puberty

Most girls (80 per cent) with pubertal development before 8 years of age have no detectable organic disease. **653** shows a 4-year-old girl with true precocious puberty. Premature thelarche (**654**) is commoner than the complete syndrome.

654

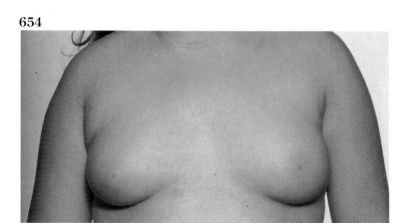

655

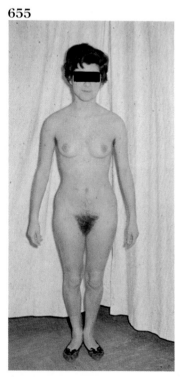

656

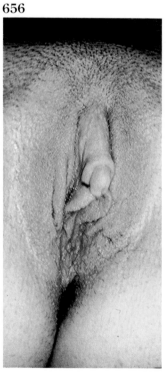

Congenital adrenal hyperplasia

Females with 21-hydroxylase and 11 ß-hydroxylase deficiency may develop some features of sexual precocity with increased muscular development (**655**). Breast development may be poor because of the increased androgen production. Pubertal changes are associated with a degree of virilisation (**656**).

Miscellaneous causes

Precocious puberty in the female (as in the male) may rarely be associated with brain tumours, hypothyroidism or polyostotic dysplasia. Ovarian (**657**) or adrenal tumours (**658** and **659**) may be associated with sexual precocity in the female.

657

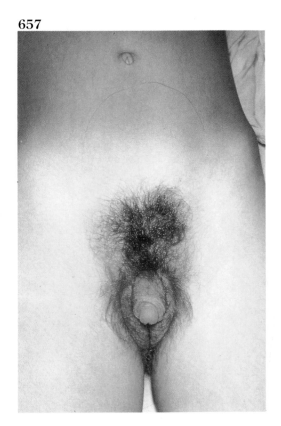

658

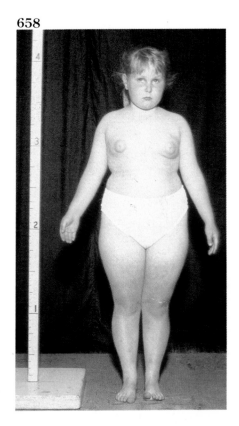

659

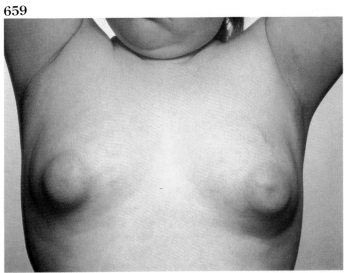

Disorders presenting as delayed puberty

Males

The onset of puberty in boys generally occurs between 10 and 16 years of age. The child or his parents will usually seek medical advice if sexual maturation has not occurred by the latter age.

Constitutional delay in puberty

The age of onset of puberty varies considerably, but is partly determined by the age of onset of puberty in the parents. The diagnosis of constitutional delay is made by exclusion if full clinical examination, serum gonadotrophins and testosterone and bone age are normal. A variant is the syndrome of apparently small genitalia in fat boys (**660**). The reduction in genital size is apparent rather than real, for the penile shaft is buried in the suprapubic fat pad and is normal in size. The testes are also normal in size for a prepubertal boy (**661**). The condition is sometimes misdiagnosed as the very rare Fröhlich's syndrome, which is caused by a hypothalamic tumour.

660

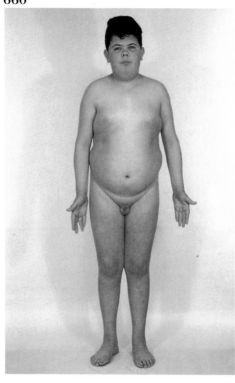

661

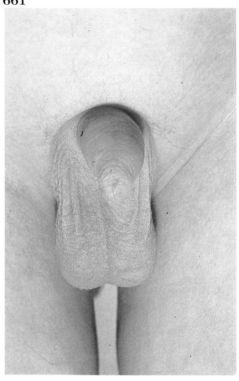

Organic causes of delay in puberty

True delay in puberty may occur as a result of hyperthalamic or pituitary disease (see page 13) or primary testicular disease. **662** shows a 21-year-old boy with hypogonadism and blindness resulting from a calcified hypothalamic tumour (**663**). **664** and **665** show an 18-year-old and 21-year-old boy with Kallmann's syndrome of hypogonadotrophic hypogonadism and anosmia. The testes are small in this condition (**666** shows the 4ml testes of the patient shown in **665**). Testicular disease causing delayed puberty may result from chromosomal disorders (see pages 142 to 146), other developmental anomalies (see pages 146 to 147) or from other testicular disease (e.g. orchitis, or as a result of the use of cytotoxic drugs). If the patient does not receive androgen therapy, secondary sexual characteristics do not develop, the skin remains fine, and fine wrinkling develops around the mouth (**667**).

662

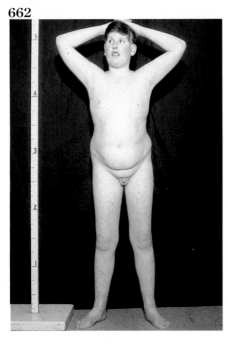

663

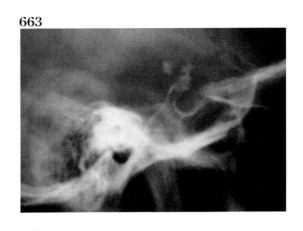

664

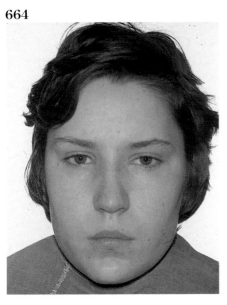

665

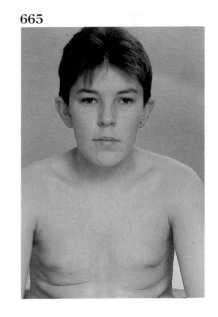

666

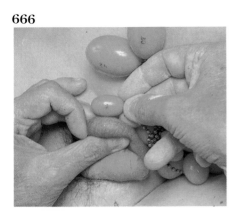

667

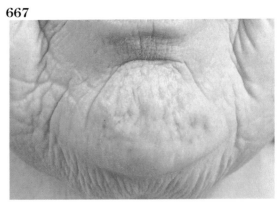

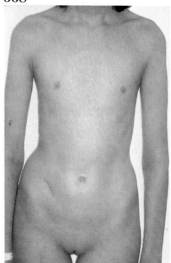

668

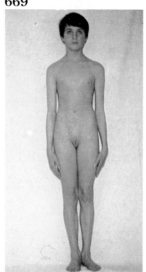

669

Females

The onset of puberty in girls generally occurs between the ages of 9 and 15 years and menstruation begins about one year later, although it may be irregular for one to two years before a regular cycle is established.

Constitutional delay in puberty

Constitutional delay in puberty in the female (**668** and **669**, seen here in an 18-year-old female), as in the male can be identified only after excluding hypothalamic, pituitary, ovarian or chromosomal disorders. The size of the ovaries (**670**) and uterus (**671**) can be assessed by ultrasound.

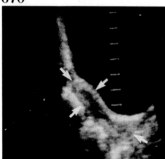

670

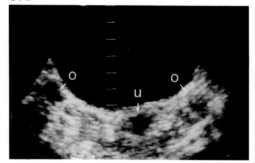

671

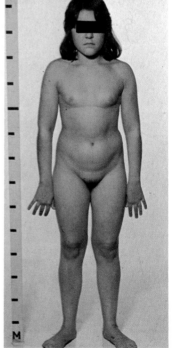

673

Organic causes of delay in puberty

True delay in puberty may result from hypothalamic or pituitary disease (see page 14) or disorders of sexual development. Prolonged primary amenorrhoea is associated with a failure to develop secondary sexual characteristics. **672** and **673** show a 21-year-old woman with Kallmann's syndrome of hypogonadotrophic hypogonadism associated with anosmia.

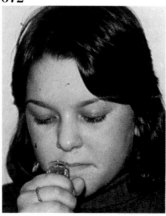

672

Disorders presenting as secondary amenorrhoea or infertility

Secondary amenorrhoea or infertility are common reasons for referral to endocrine or gynaecological clinics. It is important to remember that pregnancy is the commonest cause of secondary amenorrhoea and that all contraceptive techniques are fallible, before extensive investigation is started.

Physiological secondary amenorrhoea

The commonest cause of secondary amenorrhoea, as stated previously, is pregnancy. Periods of amenorrhoea may also be observed in the early years of menstruation, after parturition and also in the years just before the menopause.

'Functional' secondary amenorrhoea

Amenorrhoea may accompany psychological or physical stress. Psychological illness or anxiety in young women may be accompanied by temporary cessation of menstruation. Physical illness or malnutrition can have a similar effect; secondary amenorrhoea is invariably present in anorexia nervosa (**674** and **675**) and small pale atrophic ovaries may be seen at laparoscopy (**676**). Rigorous physical training schedules are frequently associated with amenorrhoea.

Hypothalamic-pituitary disease

Hypothalamic and/or pituitary disease is frequently accompanied by secondary amenorrhoea and infertility (see page 14). The presence of hyperprolactinaemia, with (**677**) or without galactorrhoea, is common and may play a major part in the suppression of ovarian function. It is not always possible to identify a cause for the galactorrhoea. A proportion of patients with 'idiopathic' galactorrhoea will ultimately develop pituitary tumours.

674

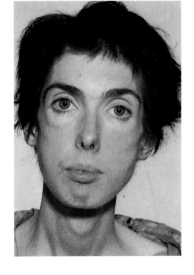

675

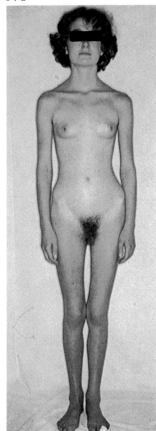

676

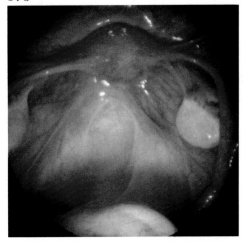

677

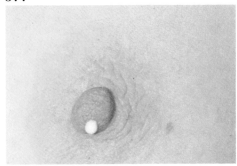

678

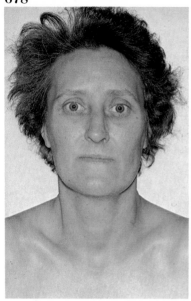

Ovarian disease

Premature ovarian failure

Premature menopause is relatively common. It is often not possible to identify a cause but it is thought to be autoimmune in origin in some patients. It may be associated with other autoimmune disorders particularly Addison's disease (**678**). The symptoms and clinical features are similar to those of the normal menopause.

Polycystic ovary syndrome

The major clinical features are obesity, amenorrhoea (or gross menstrual irregularity), hirsutism (**679** and **680**) and infertility. The ovaries are enlarged with a thickened capsule and contain multiple cysts. These are best demonstrated by ultrasound (**681**). Ovarian enlargement may also be observed during gynaecography (**682**) and at laparotomy (**683**). The characteristic appearance on section is shown in **684**. (**681** is reproduced by permission of the editors of *Therapeutic Applications of LHRH*, RSM Services International Congress and Symposium series, 1986; **105**: 77–84.)

679

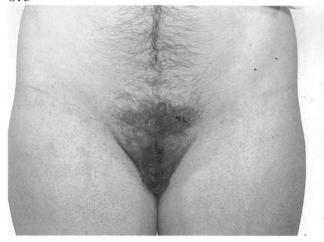

680

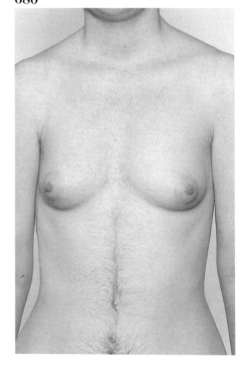

681

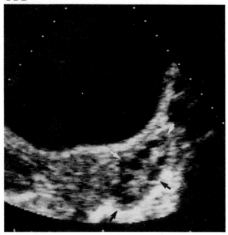

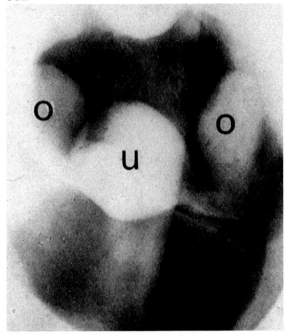

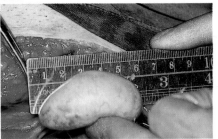

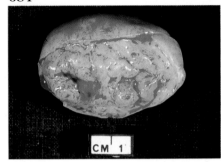

Ovarian hyperthecosis syndrome

This is probably a variant of the polycystic ovary syndrome. The clinical features of the syndromes are indistinguishable but the ovaries are relatively smaller and do not contain cysts. An excess of thecal cells is present in the ovarian stroma.

Masculinising ovarian tumours

These tumours are rare. Amenorrhoea occurs early in the clinical course. Virilisation with coarsening of the skin, hirsutism (685) breast atrophy and clitoral hypertrophy (686) develop with time.

Other causes

Secondary amenorrhoea and reduced fertility may also be seen in some other endocrine disorders (e.g. Cushing's syndrome and hyperthyroidism), serious organic disease or after treatment with certain drugs (e.g. oral contraceptives, phenothiazines, tricyclic anti-depressants and some antihypertensives). Simple obesity may also be associated with secondary amenorrhoea without any evident endocrine disorder.

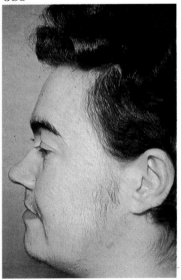

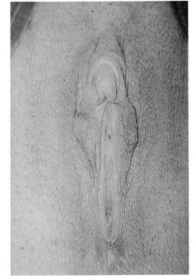

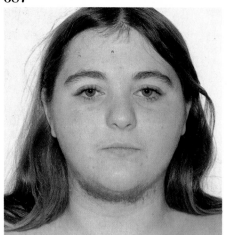

687

Disorders presenting as hirsutism or virilism

Hirsutism cannot be defined objectively. The complaint of hirsutism by the patient is always an indication for physical examination, and investigation if the physician feels the degree of hirsutism falls outside the wide range of normality. There is considerable physiological variation between individuals, families and ethnic groups. The location of the excess hair may vary considerably, occurring below the chin (**687** and **688**) or elsewhere on the face (**689** and **690**), round the nipples (**691**) over the lower back (**692**) or on the limbs. Significant organic disease causing hirsutism is almost invariably associated with amenorrhoea.

688

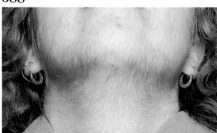

690

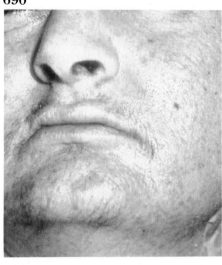

689

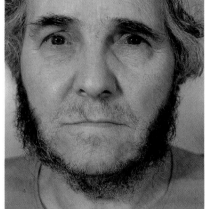

692

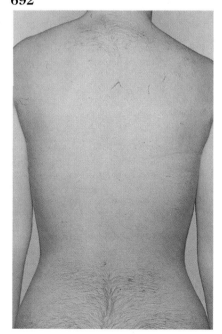

691

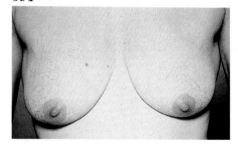

Virilisation is defined as the presence of some or all of the following features:

- Frontal baldness (**693** and **694**, from an arrhenoblastoma)
- Deepening of the voice
- Breast atrophy
- Masculine habitus (**695** and **696**, here caused by an ovarian tumour)
- Clitoral hypertrophy

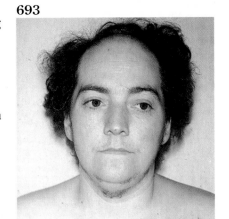

693

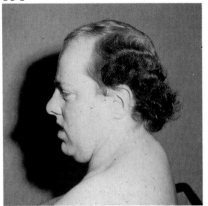

694

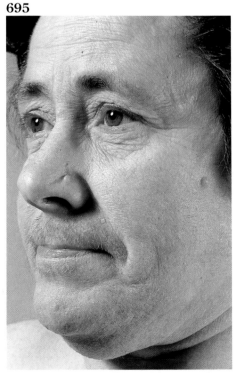

695

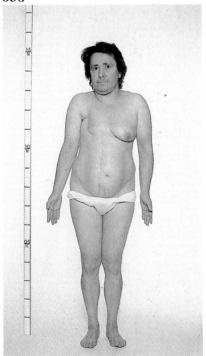

696

697

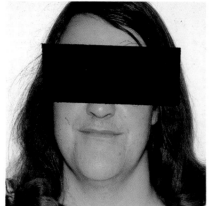

The causes of hirsutism and virilism have been covered in other sections:

- Adrenal
  Cushing's syndrome (page 126)
  Adrenal tumours (page 129)
  Congenital adrenal hyperplasia (**697** and **698**, page 137)
- Ovarian
  Polycystic ovary syndrome (page 168)
  Ovarian hyperthecosis syndrome (page 169)
  Masculinising tumours (page 169)
- Drugs
  Androgens
  Glucocorticoids
  Phenytoin
- Secondary to carcinoma (generally of bronchial origin)
  Hypertrichosis lanuginosa (**699** and **700**) — this condition remits
  with successful treatment of the tumour)

It is not possible to identify a cause of hirsutism in some patients.

698

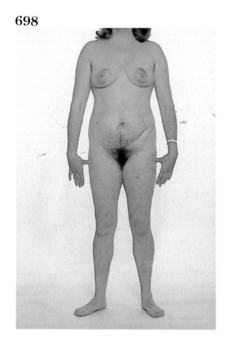

699

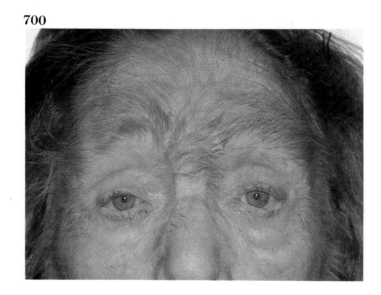

700

Chapter 6
Disorders of the breast

Introduction

In the male the breast normally remains quiescent throughout life, apart from the minor degree of physiological enlargement seen in most boys at puberty. In the female enlargement of the breast at puberty is followed by cyclical changes related to the menstrual cycle and secretory activity in response to pregnancy and suckling. Hormonal influences on the breast are complex and not completely understood; the dominant effects result from oestrogens, progesterone, prolactin, human placental lactogen and growth hormone, while minor effects can be attributed to thyroid hormones and corticosteroids. The breast can respond in only a limited number of ways to pathological processes — by enlargement, atrophy or milk secretion.

Disorders of the male breast

Enlargement of breast tissue occurs in most boys at an early stage during the development of puberty. Enlargement may be unilateral (**701**) or bilateral (**702**) and is only occasionally sufficiently prominent to cause embarrassment (**703**).

701

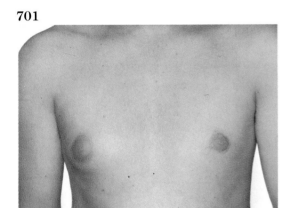

702

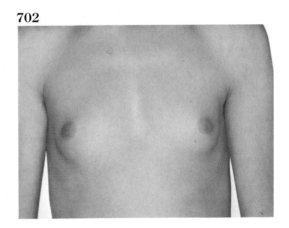

703

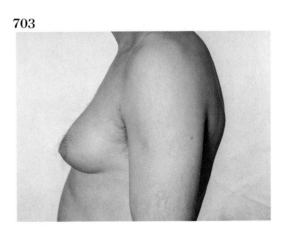

Puberty gynaecomastia should not be confused with the fatty swelling of the breast region seen in any obese male (**704**). In obesity it is not possible to palpate glandular tissue when the hand is applied firmly to the breast and pressed against the chest wall. The appearance of gynaecomastia can be aggravated by the presence of pectus excavatum (**705**). An abscess may result from local trauma and cause unilateral gynaecomastia (**706**). Oestrogen ingestion (e.g. in the course of treatment for prostatic carcinoma) or production by tumours can cause gynaecomastia (**707** and **708** show breast enlargement in a 50-year-old man with an oestrogen-secreting adreno-cortical carcinoma). When gynaecomastia is marked (**709** and **710**) the possibility of Klinefelter's syndrome should be considered (**711**). The very small firm testes (**712**) associated with this condition are usually easily differentiated from the larger testes of a normal boy entering puberty (see also pages 142 to 143).

704

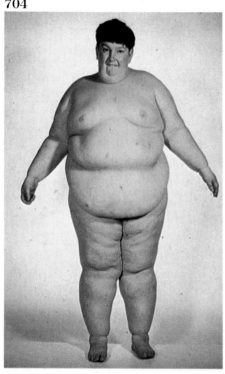

705

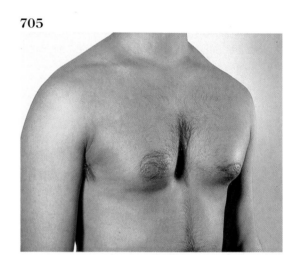

706

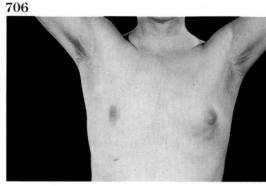

707

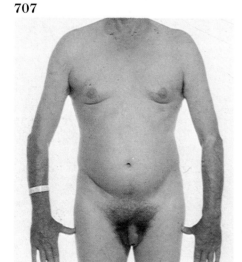

708

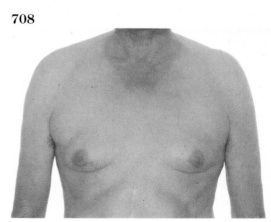

709

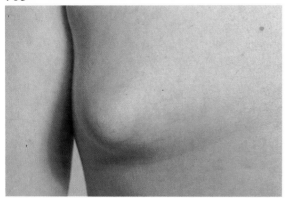

710

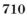
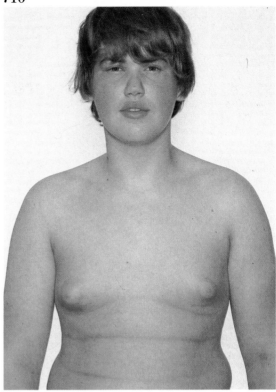

711

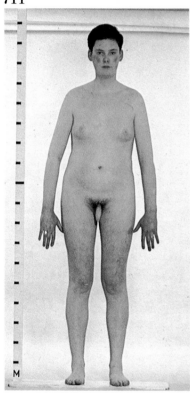

712

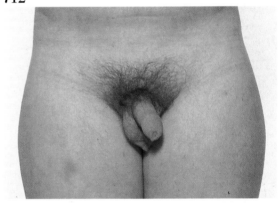

713

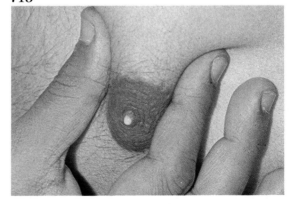

Secretion from the male breast may occur in several conditions. Brown secretion may be seen in men treated with anabolic steroids for aplastic anaemia. True galactorrhoea in men (**713**) can result from any of the conditions causing this in females, particularly hyperprolactinaemic states resulting from drugs, hypothalamic-pituitary disease or from the lactogenic action of growth hormone in acromegaly (see page 23).

Disorders of the female breast

These disorders may be congenital or acquired. Congenital absence of breast tissue is usually associated with poor development of the pectoralis major (**714**), but may also indicate a chromosomal anomaly. **715** shows lack of breast development in a 17-year-old phenotypic female with gonadal dysgenesis and a 46,XY karyotype. In Turner's syndrome the nipples are poorly developed and widely spaced and the breasts are usually atrophic (**716**).

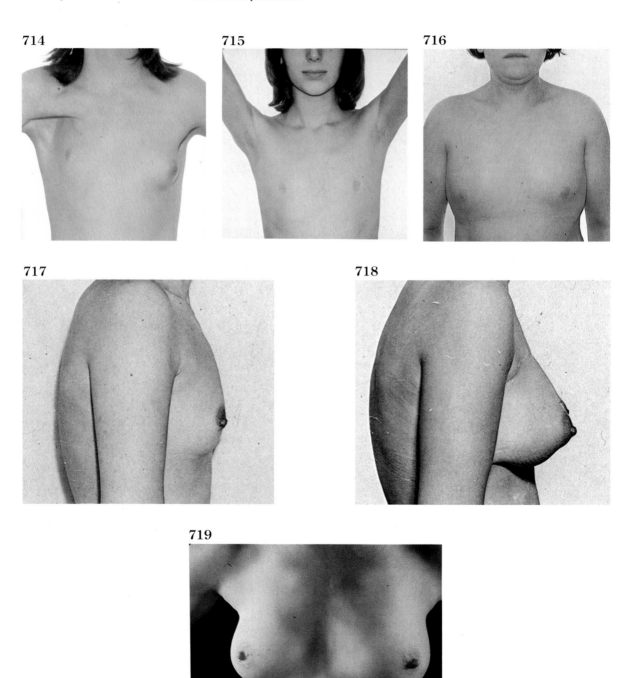

714

715

716

717

718

719

Small breasts usually represent the lower end of the normal range and do not preclude normal suckling. Secondary atrophy of the breasts may occur without evident cause or may follow a period of weight loss. The improvement in appearance following enhancement procedures (e.g. silastic implants) is usually mirrored by a dramatic psychological improvement. **717** and **718** show breast atrophy and the result after insertion of silastic implants. Asymmetrical breasts are common but this is rarely so marked as to cause concern (**719**).

720

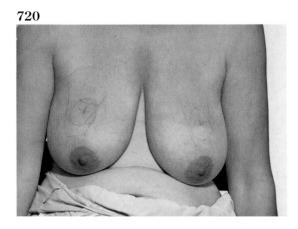

721

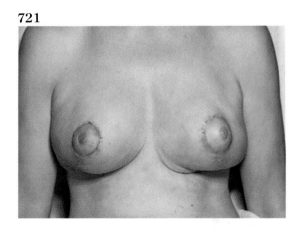

722

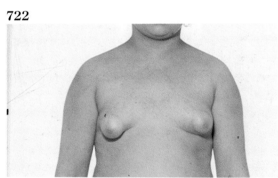

723

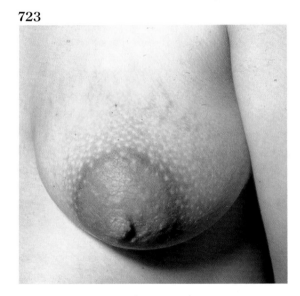

Unduly large breasts may occur as a primary phenomenon or they may develop in adult life without any obvious cause (**720** and **721** show a patient with large breasts before and after plastic surgery). Obesity is usually accompanied by deposition of fat in the breasts which diminishes with weight reduction. Apparent overgrowth of the areolae is common during puberty (**722**) and gradually recedes as full breast development occurs. Stimulation of the nipple causes contraction of the local musculature and a more normal appearance is restored. Pigmentation of the nipples is a physiological occurrence during pregnancy but may be marked (**723**).

Non-physiological secretion of milk from the breasts is a relatively common endocrine problem. A woman may not be aware of the secretion and expression of the breast is part of the routine endocrine examination of all women with infertility, amenorrhoea, hirsutism and suspected hypothalamic-pituitary disease. The causes of galactorrhoea are discussed on pages 30 and 31. Duct ectasia, shown here on mammography (**724** and **725**), is a cause of breast secretion in women with a normal prolactin level. Brown or blood-stained secretion should alert the clinician to the possibility of a breast tumour. Tumours of the breast are outside the range of this book.

724

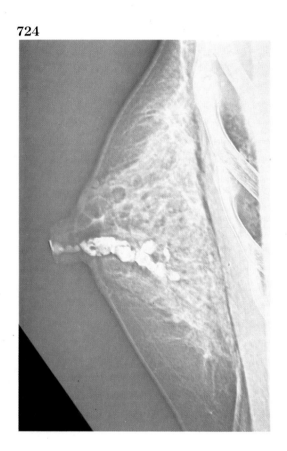

725

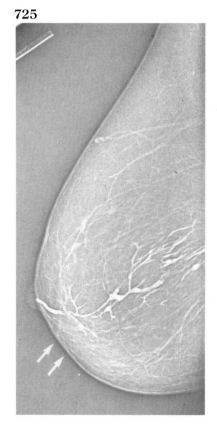

Chapter 7
Diabetes mellitus

Introduction

Diabetes mellitus is the term given to a syndrome which has as its most prominent feature elevation of the blood glucose, frequently associated with glycosuria. The elevation of the blood glucose may be entirely asymptomatic, but glycosuria causes an osmotic diuresis with polyuria, secondary polydipsia and is generally accompanied by weight loss. The hyperglycaemia of diabetes results from abnormalities of insulin secretion or action. Insulin is secreted by the pancreatic B cells of the islets of Langerhans which make up approximately 80 per cent of the islet cell mass. The other cell types secrete glucagon (A cells), somatostatin (D cells) and pancreatic polypeptide. Insulin secretion is modified by other hormones (e.g. glucagon and somatostatin) and by a number of metabolic factors. Insulin secretion in diabetes may be deficient, delayed or otherwise inappropriate for the prevailing blood glucose level, or its action may be affected by circulating antagonists (e.g. antibodies) or by abnormalities of the tissue receptors.

Classification of diabetes mellitus

Hereditary idiopathic diabetes mellitus

Subclinical

a) Prediabetes or potential diabetes where there is no abnormality of carbohydrate metabolism even after steroid administration, but the individual is at risk for the future development of the condition

b) Latent diabetes refers to normal individuals who develop impairment of carbohydrate metabolism in response to stress or steroids

c) Chemical diabetes refers to patients with glycosuria, hyperglycaemia and impaired carbohydrate intolerance who are asymptomatic. Approximately 2 to 4 per cent of this group will develop diabetes each year

Clinical (overt) diabetes

a) Insulin-dependent diabetes mellitus (IDDM) — otherwise known as juvenile onset diabetes or Type I diabetes

b) Non-insulin-dependent diabetes mellitus (NIDDM) — otherwise known as maturity onset diabetes or Type II diabetes

Malnutrition-related diabetes mellitus (MRDM)

a) Fibrocalculous pancreatic diabetes (FCPD) — associated with severe malnutrition and exocrine pancreatic deficiency. This form is found in south-east Asia, the Indian subcontinent and South America

b) Protein-deficient pancreatic diabetes — otherwise known as J-type diabetes and first described in Jamaica

Secondary to pancreatic disease

After acute or chronic pancreatitis
After pancreatectomy
Haemochromatosis
Tumours
After removal of an islet cell tumour (usually transient)
Cystic fibrosis

Secondary to other endocrine disorders

Cushing's syndrome
Acromegaly
Phaeochromocytoma
Hyperthyroidism
Aldosteronism
Glucagonoma
Laron dwarfism

Precipitated by drugs

Thiazide diuretics and diazoxide
Corticosteroids
Oral contraceptives
Phenothiazines

Insulin receptor abnormalities

Congenital lipodystrophy
Anti-receptor antibodies

Inherited disorders

Type I glycogen storage disease
DIDMOAD syndrome
Ataxia telangiectasia syndrome
Werner's syndrome
Down's syndrome
Turner's syndrome
Lipoatrophic dystrophies

Related to non-endocrine disease

Chronic renal failure
Liver disease

Clinical features of diabetes mellitus

Other than the sequelae of hyperglycaemia — polyuria, polydipsia, fatigue, anorexia and weight loss — the clinical features of diabetes mellitus are those of its acute or chronic complications (which may be specific to idiopathic diabetes or secondary to the metabolic disorders) and/or those of any underlying cause. Non-insulin-dependent diabetes is frequently associated with obesity.

Features of pancreatic diseases causing diabetes mellitus

Chronic pancreatitis with calcification (MRDM) is a rare cause of diabetes except in certain areas such as southern India. **726** and **727** show pancreatic calcification. Haemochromatosis may be recognised by the characteristic bronze pigmentation (**728**) caused by deposits of haemosiderin and melanin, and also the associated hepatosplenomegaly related to the cirrhosis.

726

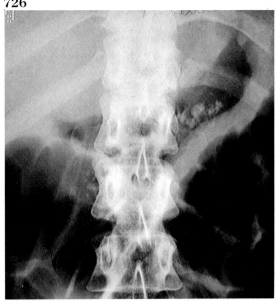

727

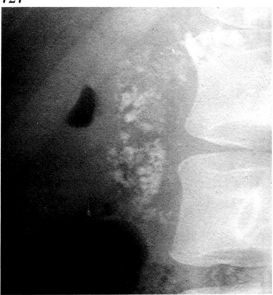

728

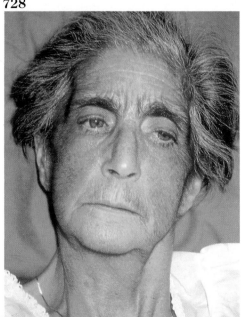

Features of other endocrine diseases causing diabetes mellitus

Cushing's syndrome (**729**) caused by pituitary or adrenal disease or as a result of steroid administration is commonly complicated by diabetes mellitus. Acromegaly (**730**) is associated with overt or subclinical diabetes in at least one-quarter of cases, although this rarely causes any problems in management. Phaeo-chromocytomas may lead to diabetes (**731** shows an mIBG scan). Hyperthyroidism (**732**) from any cause may precipitate diabetes in pre-diabetic or latent diabetic individuals. The condition usually remits with effective antithyroid therapy. These disorders are described in greater detail elsewhere in the book.

729

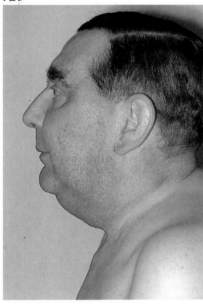

730

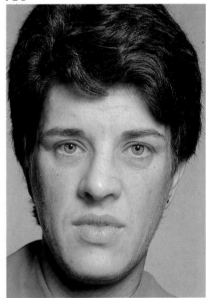

731

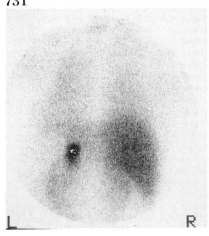

732

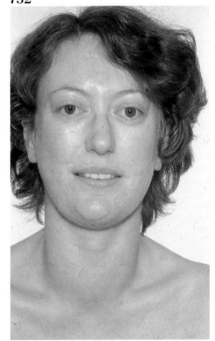

Features of non-endocrine disease causing diabetes mellitus

Carbohydrate tolerance is impaired in most patients with chronic renal failure (**733** shows a patient with a characteristic uraemic appearance). Chronic liver disease may also be associated with diabetes. **734** shows a patient with ascites caused by hepatic cirrhosis who developed diabetes.

733

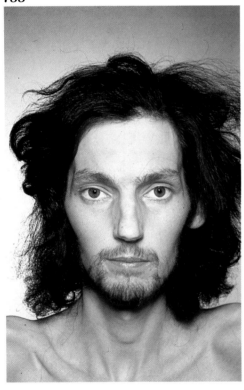

734

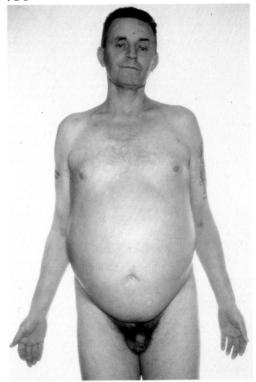

Complications of diabetes mellitus

Acute complications

The acute complications of diabetes are shown in
735. The most important of these are:

- Insulin allergy
- Hyperlipidaemia
- Hypoglycaemia
- Diabetic ketoacidaemia (**736** shows the dry tongue of a dehydrated diabetic with this condition)
- Lactic acidaemia
- Hyperosmolar non-ketotic diabetic coma
- Acute infections
- Acute neuropathy

735

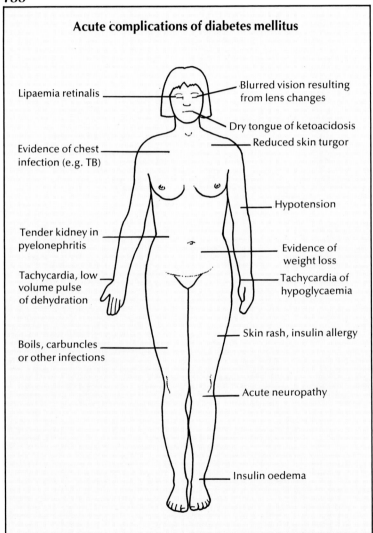

Acute complications of diabetes mellitus

Lipaemia retinalis

Blurred vision resulting
from lens changes

Dry tongue of ketoacidosis

Reduced skin turgor

Evidence of chest
infection (e.g. TB)

Hypotension

Tender kidney in
pyelonephritis

Evidence of
weight loss

Tachycardia, low
volume pulse
of dehydration

Tachycardia of
hypoglycaemia

Skin rash, insulin allergy

Boils, carbuncles
or other infections

Acute neuropathy

Insulin oedema

736

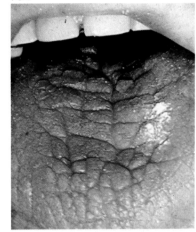

Insulin allergy

This condition is uncommon (particularly with highly purified insulins), and erythema at the injection site is usually caused by either contaminants or infection (**737**). The usual general manifestations are erythema (**738**), urticaria (**739** and **740**) and delayed allergic reactions (**741**) but severe anaphylactic shock may occur. These problems can be avoided by using human insulin preparations. Desensitisation can be undertaken in true insulin allergy but this is rarely required.

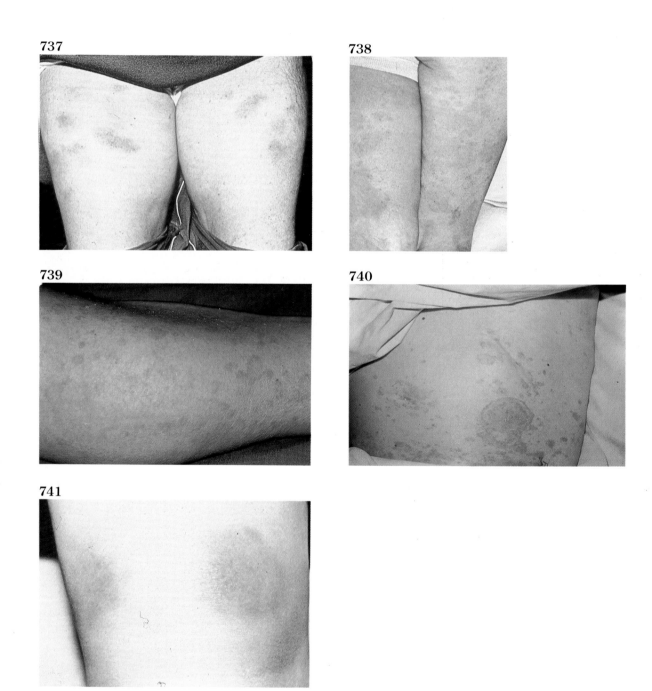

737

738

739

740

741

Hyperlipidaemia

In diabetic ketoacidosis the serum may appear milky as a result of severe hyperlipidaemia (**742**). Lipaemia retinalis (**743**) may be seen in the optic fundi.

742

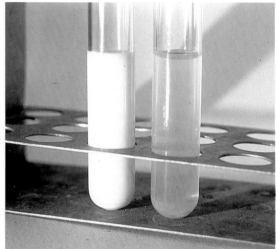

743

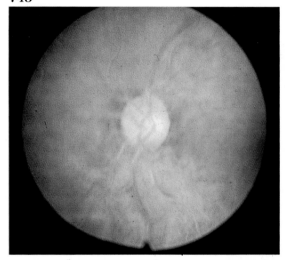

Acute infection

Acute bacterial infections may affect the skin causing boils or carbuncles (**744**), or the urinary tract. Candidal infections of the mouth, such as angular stomatitis (**745**), or more generalised infection of the buccal cavity may occur (**746** shows candidiasis in a denture wearer). Candidal infections may also occur in the genital region leading to balanitis (**747**) or vulvitis (**748**), and the infection may spread to the upper inner thighs (**749**) and skin flexures leading to severe intertrigo (**750**).

744

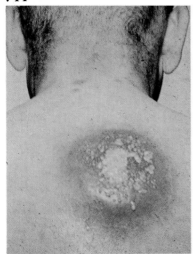

745

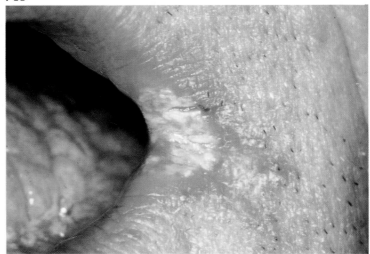

746

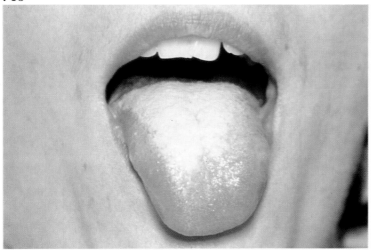

747

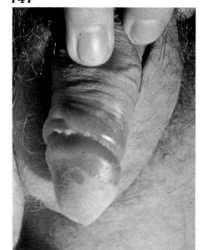

748

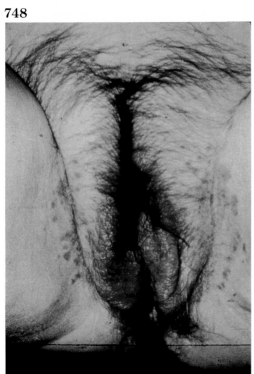

749

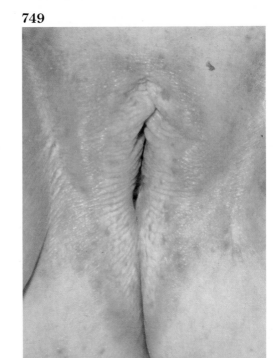

750

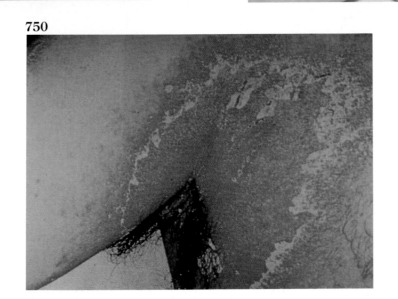

Acute neuropathy

Acute neuropathy may be seen during or after a period of poor diabetic control. A variety of neuropathic syndromes may be seen affecting motor and sensory nerves in lower and upper limbs, including mononeuritis multiplex. **751** shows bilateral ulnar nerve palsies in a diabetic. Diabetic amyotrophy is caused by a proximal radiculopathy. Wasting of proxi-mal limb muscles, particularly the thighs (**752**), is common and upper motor neurone lesions may also be present. Isolated cranial nerve palsies, e.g. of the IIIrd nerve may occur (**753** and **754**), although the pupil is usually spared in diabetic IIIrd nerve palsy.

751

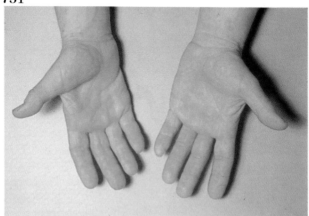

752

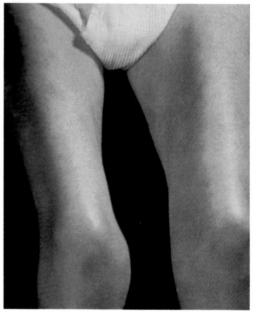

753

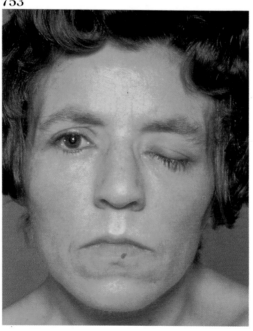

754

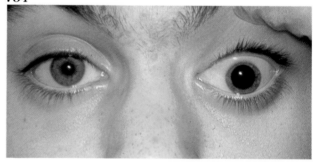

Chronic complications

The chronic complications of diabetes are noted in **755**. The most important of these are:

- Insulin lipodystrophy
  Hypertrophy
  Atrophy
- Fibrosis at injection sites
- Atherosclerosis and hypertension
- Renal disease
- Chronic neuropathy
- Ophthalmic disease
  Disturbance of visual acuity
  Cataracts
  Iridopathy
  Retinopathy and maculopathy

- Dermatological disease
  Bacterial infections (v.s.)
  Candidiasis (v.s.)
  Acanthosis nigricans
  Diabetic dermopathy
  Necrobiosis lipoidica
  Granuloma annulare
  Subcutaneous lipid deposits
  Xanthoma diabeticorum
- Chronic infections
- Diabetic foot disease and osteopathy
- Fetal abnormalities
  Malformations
  Growth retardation
  Macrosomia
- Musculoskeletal problems
  Dupuytren's contracture

The major organ and tissue changes of diabetes are also classified as those caused by microvascular disease and those caused by macrovascular disease. The importance of this distinction is that the microvascular complications giving rise to retinopathy, neuropathy and nephropathy are generally specific for diabetes, while the macrovascular complications are similar to those seen in non-diabetics although they occur more frequently in diabetics.

755

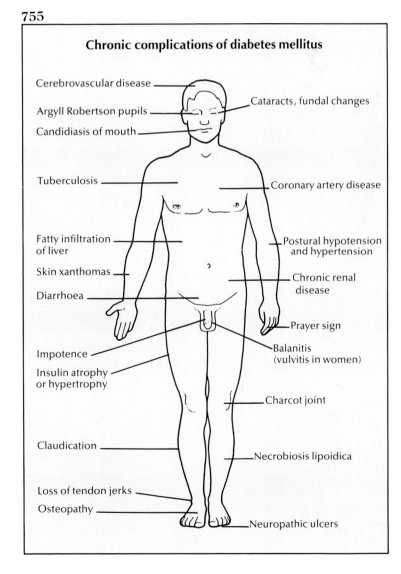

Chronic complications of diabetes mellitus

Cerebrovascular disease
Argyll Robertson pupils
Candidiasis of mouth
Cataracts, fundal changes
Tuberculosis
Coronary artery disease
Fatty infiltration of liver
Postural hypotension and hypertension
Skin xanthomas
Diarrhoea
Chronic renal disease
Prayer sign
Impotence
Balanitis (vulvitis in women)
Insulin atrophy or hypertrophy
Charcot joint
Claudication
Necrobiosis lipoidica
Loss of tendon jerks
Osteopathy
Neuropathic ulcers

Insulin lipodystrophy

This occurs at the site of insulin injections. The hypertrophy consists of soft lipomatous swellings caused by an increase in total lipid and hypertrophied fat cells (**756** and **757**). The condition is common in those under the age of 20 years. Atrophy is caused by loss of fatty tissue (**758** and **759**). Atrophy and hypertrophy may be seen in adjacent areas in the same patient (**760**). It may improve spontaneously or after the injection of neutral highly purified insulin into the affected area.

757

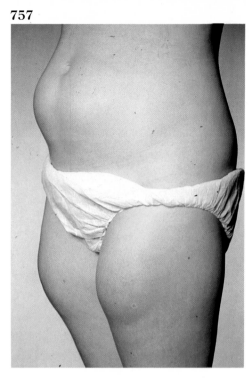

756

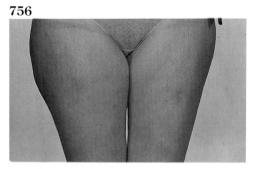

758

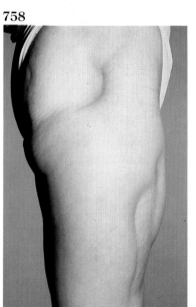

759

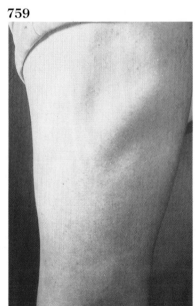

760

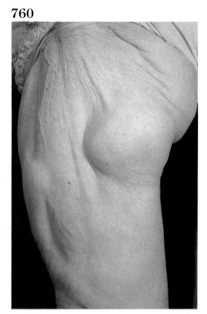

761

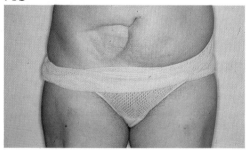

Fibrosis at injection sites

This can often be detected only by palpation. It results from over-frequent injection at a single or a limited number of sites (**761**). This is often favoured by the patient as it is less painful, but it may give rise to considerable management problems as it leads to variability in the rate of insulin absorption.

Atherosclerosis

This appears earlier and is more extensive in diabetics than non-diabetics. The distribution of the disease is essentially similar to that seen in non-diabetics. Limb vessel involvement may lead to intermittent claudication or gangrene (**762** and **763**), such lesions being particularly prone to infection in the diabetic, often with surrounding cellulitis (**764** and **765**) which may be extensive. An underlying osteitis may be revealed radiologically (**766**). Local amputation can yield good results (**767**). Involvement of other vessels may lead to premature coronary artery or cerebrovascular disease. Myocardial infarction is the commonest cause of death in diabetes and hypertension is common. Atherosclerosis may also play a significant part in some of the other complications of diabetes — namely glomerulosclerosis, retinopathy and neuropathy.

762

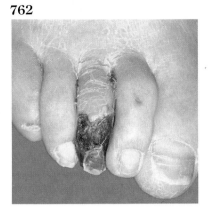

763

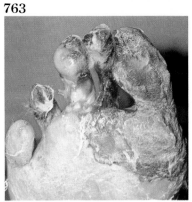

764

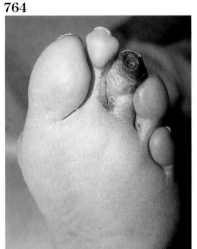

765

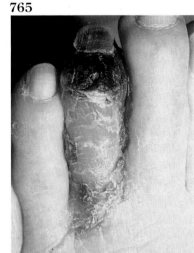

766

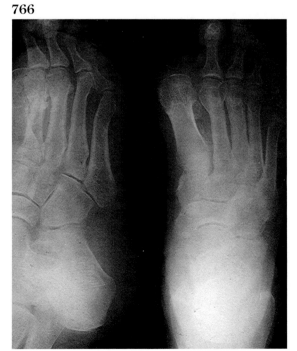

767

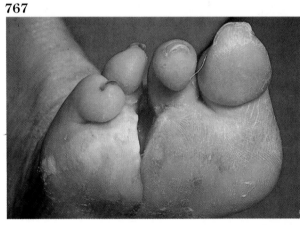

Atherosclerosis must be distinguished from the specific and characteristic vascular lesion of diabetes, the microangiopathy which is mainly responsible for the nephropathy, retinopathy and neuropathy as well as some of the skin lesions. The specific basement membrane thickening of diabetic microangiopathy may affect all arterioles, venules and capillaries to a greater or lesser extent.

Renal disease

Renal complications may be non-specific, for example, caused by pyelonephritis (**768** shows a pyelogram with loss of the renal cortex and clubbing of the calyces), nephrosclerosis or hypertension. Severe infection can lead to a necrotising papillitis. The specific diabetic renal lesion is diabetic glomerulosclerosis giving rise to Kimmelstiel–Wilson syndrome. This may lead to nephrotic syndrome with facial and generalised oedema (**769** shows pitting oedema in nephrotic syndrome).

768

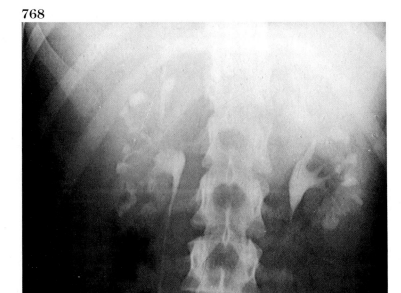

769

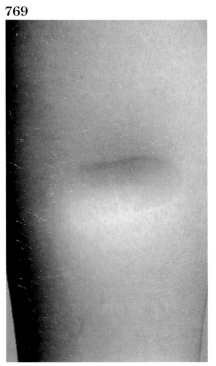

Chronic neuropathy

This condition results from a combination of atherosclerosis and microangiopathy. It may comprise the following:

a) Sensory nerve involvement which is generally distal in distribution and may lead to trophic ulceration (**770** and **771**), which may be complicated by infection (**772** and **773**) and a neuropathic arthropathy — a Charcot joint (**774** and **775**).

b) Motor nerve involvement causing muscle weakness and wasting. This is generally proximal in distribution.

c) Mixed syndromes — mononeuritis multiplex or a mixed peripheral neuropathy.

d) Autonomic nerve involvement causing pupillary changes (Argyll Robertson pupils), dependent oedema, reduced sweating, bowel, bladder and sphincter disturbances, reduced potency and postural hypotension.

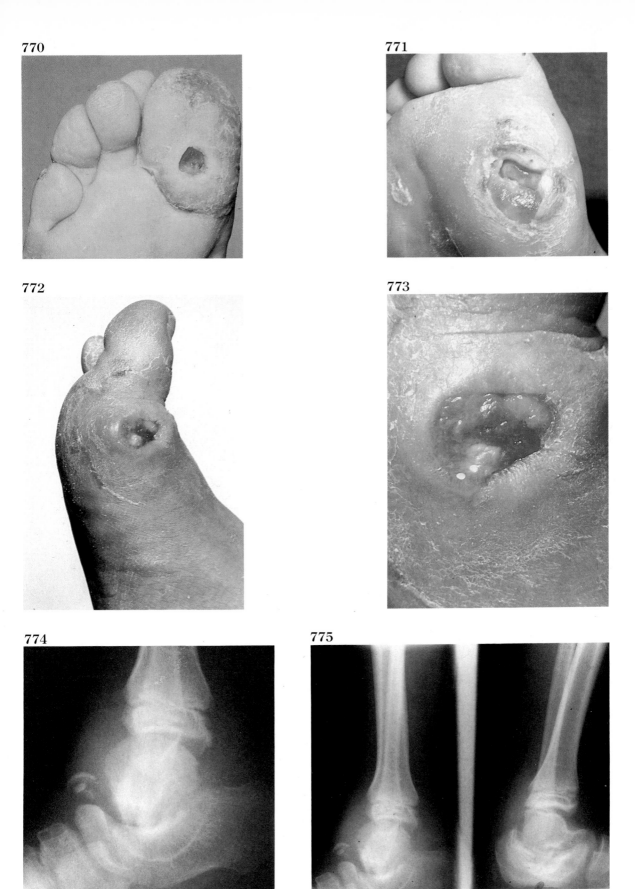

Disturbances of visual acuity. These disturbances are common in young diabetics with widely fluctuating blood sugar levels, and are largely caused by differences in osmotic pressure between the lens and the extracellular fluid.

Cataracts (776 and 777). The cataracts specifically caused by diabetes are rare but can occur in young patients. They are usually bilateral and are associated with poor metabolic control. They have a snowflake appearance and occur in the subcapsular region of the lens. Senile cataracts occur more frequently and at an earlier age in diabetics

Iridopathy. This condition is seen in some poorly treated younger diabetics where glycogen is deposited in the pigmented epithelium of the posterior surface of the iris. Later a meshwork of new blood vessels develops over the anterior surface of the iris, eventually encircling the pupil. Repeated haemorrhage into the anterior chamber leads to glaucoma which is the final result of the process. Open angle glaucoma is also more common in diabetics, although the reason for this is not clear.

776

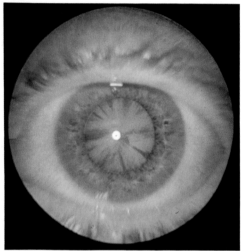

777

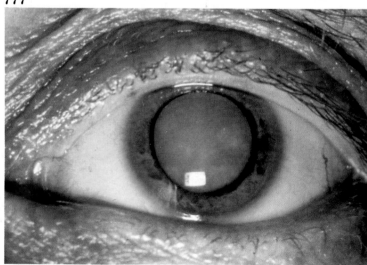

Retinopathy. This may be non-specific resulting from hypertensive or atherosclerotic changes, or may be specific resulting from diabetic microangiopathy. **778** shows a normal retina for comparison. The lesions of diabetic retinopathy are:

a)   *Venous changes* consisting initially of generalised dilatation of veins (**779** shows venous dilatation and also microaneurysms within circinate hard exudates); later beading, tortuosity, varicosities and sheathing (**780**) may occur.

b)   *Arterial changes* consisting of hyalinisation and narrowing of the arteries (**781** shows hyalinisation of vessels and also choroidoretinitis). These changes also result in part from atherosclerosis.

778

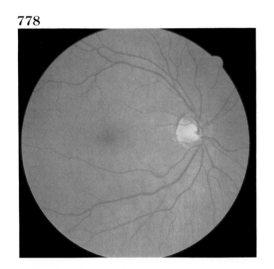

779

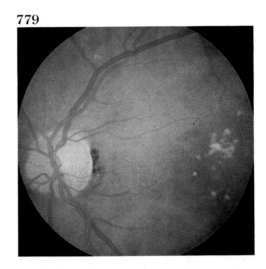

780

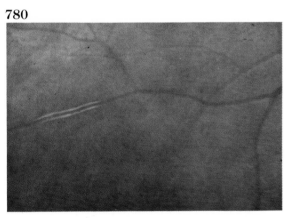

781

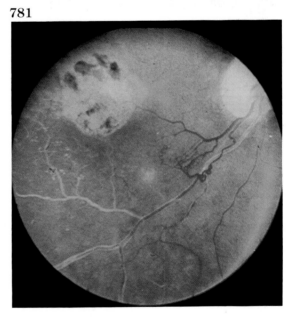

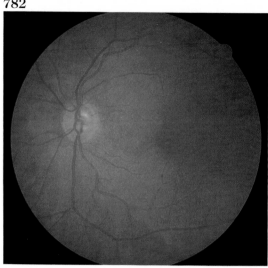

c) *Microaneurysms*. These are the characteristic feature of diabetic retinopathy. They resemble punctate haemorrhages of variable size most frequently scattered through the posterior pole and in the macular region. **782** shows microaneurysms alone, **783** associated with exudates and venous dilatation, and **784** with dot and blot haemorrhages. Fluorescence angiograms usually reveal many more microaneurysms than can be seen on routine fundoscopic examination (**785** and **786**). The presence of microaneurysms alone is the first specific change of early background retinopathy.

783

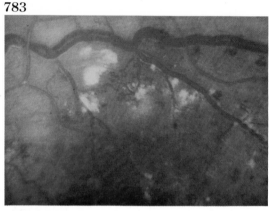

784

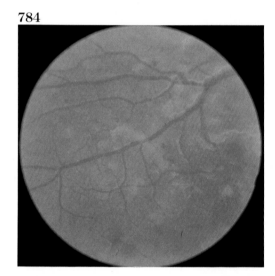

785

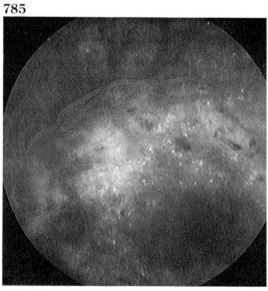

786

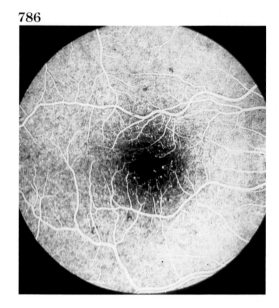

d) *Haemorrhages.* In a diabetic retina these are generally red, large, diffuse and larger than microaneurysms. **787** shows dot and blot haemorrhages and exudates, and **788** a pre-retinal smudge haemorrhage on the retinal surface below the disc. **789** shows two large flat-topped sub-hyaloid haemorrhages. Fluorescence angiography can be used to demonstrate that such haemorrhages are pre-retinal (i.e. front of the retinal vessels) as they mask the intravasular fluorescein (**790**).

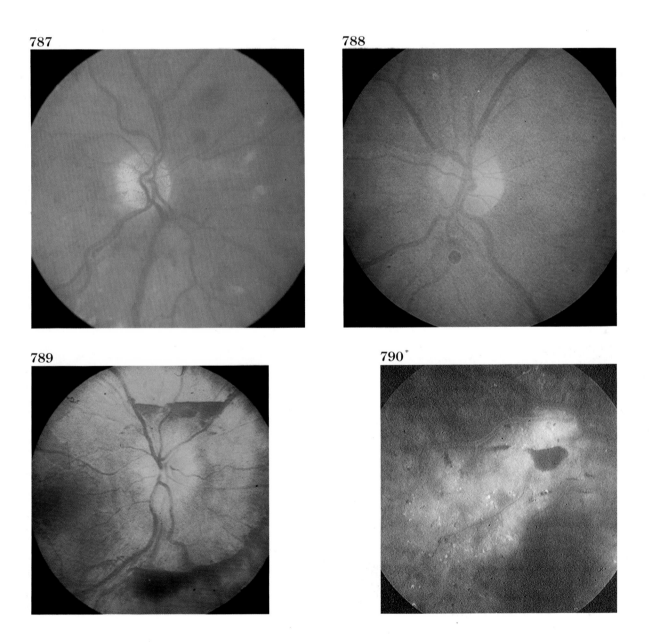

787

788

789

790˙

e) *Exudates*. These are usually hard and white or yellowish in colour. They are composed of lipid and are usually benign. **791** and **792** show a circinate retinopathy with hard exudates located in the area of the macula. **793** shows circinate exudates with corresponding angiogram and **794** a typical diabetic background retinopathy with large exudates and microaneurysms.

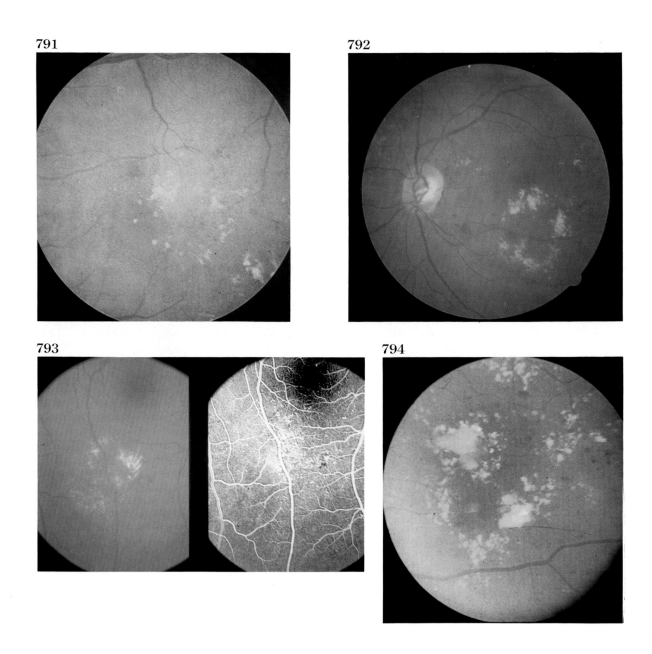

791

792

793

794

f) *Cotton wool spots*. These are retinal infarcts resulting from arterial occlusion (**795**) and are a bad prognostic sign. They are contrasted here with a number of hard exudates. The two processes are relatively independent, with random scattering of the cotton wool spots over the circinate pattern.

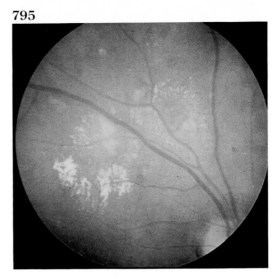

g) *Macular disease*. This is an important cause of blindness in diabetics. Exudates, microaneurysms or haemorrhages may all contribute to macular disease, but the major cause of visual impairment is macular oedema (**796**) shown here associated with multiple exudates.

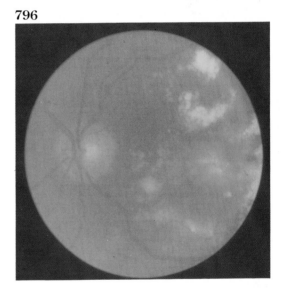

h) *Proliferative retinopathy.* This most commonly occurs in patients with widespread retinal changes (**797**). The formation of new vessels is a serious feature of diabetic retinopathy. They may arise from the disc (**798** to **800**), may mimic papilloedema (**801**), and may also arise from other areas of the retina (**802**), extend forward into the vitreous (**803** and **804**) or involve the macula. Haemorrhage is frequent (**805** and **806**) leading to fibrosis (**807**), distortion of the vitreous and tearing of the retina (v.s.).

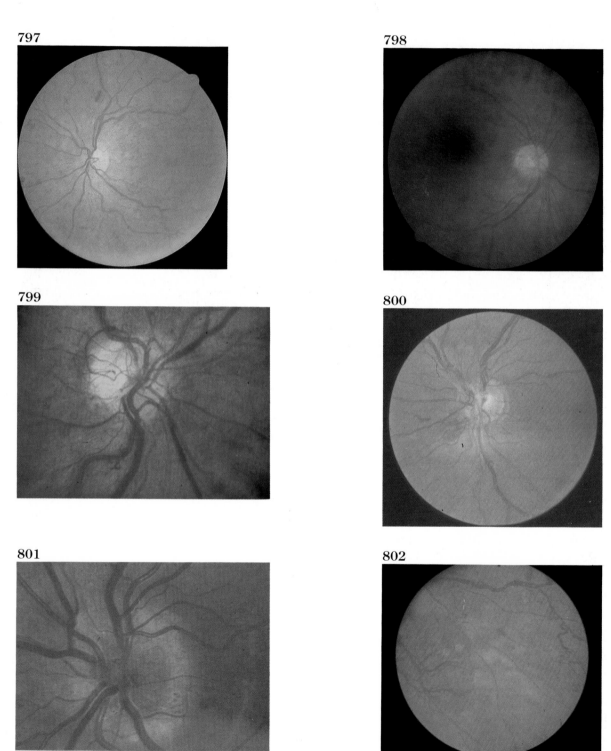

797

798

799

800

801

802

803

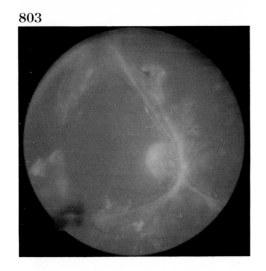

804

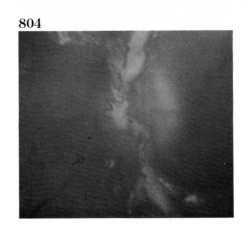

805

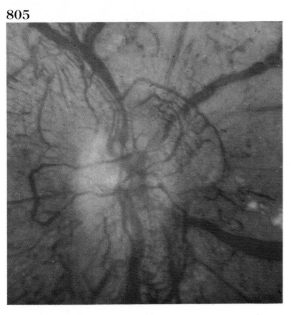

806

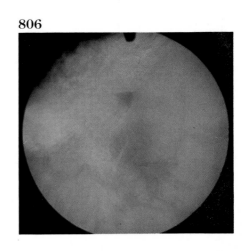

807

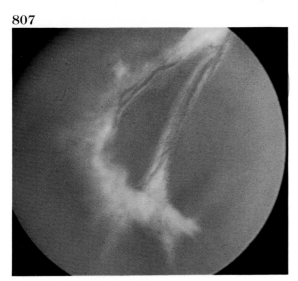

i) *Vitreous haemorrhages*. These occur from new vessels as part of the proliferative retinopathy of diabetes. They appear as a haze or a red or black reflex on fundoscopy (**808** and **809**). Later, fibrosis may lead to retinal detachment. **810** shows traction of the retina into the vitreous after organisation of a vitreous haemorrhage and contraction of the resultant connective tissue. Vitreous haemorrhages absorb and may form vitreous floaters.

808

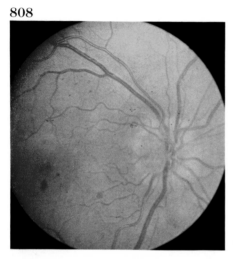

809

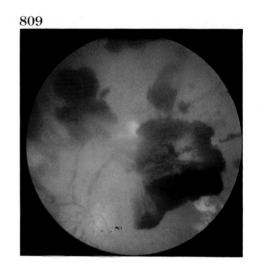

810

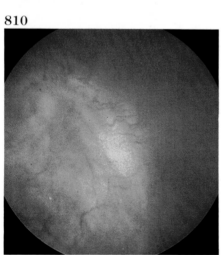

Classification of diabetic retinopathy. Patients are classified according to the changes present in the more severely affected eye. Malignant retinopathy includes those with preretinal haemorrhages, new vessel formation, fibrous proliferation or secondary glaucoma. Simple retinopathy consists of micro-aneurysms, retinal haemorrhages and exudates.

Effects of treatment. Photocoagulation produces an iatrogenic choroidoretinitis with a characteristic appearance. Laser burns are seen as white or yellow patches on the retina (**811** to **813**). Clofibrate may reduce the number of exudates. Hypophysectomy by surgery or yttrium-90 can sometimes cause a dramatic improvement in retinopathy.

811

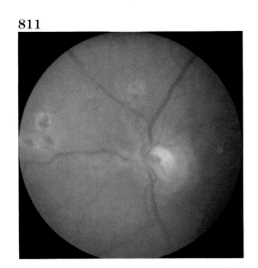

812

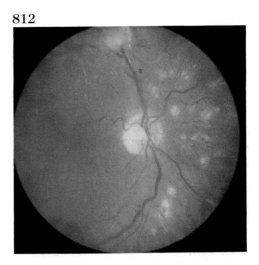

813

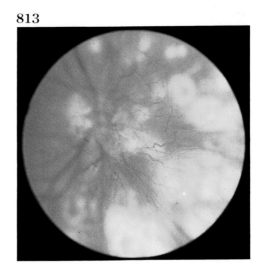

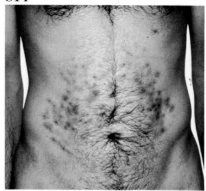

814

Dermatological disease

Pyogenic infections. These conditions are common: boils, furunculosis (**814**) and carbuncles from staphylococcal infection are a feature of poorly controlled diabetes.

Candidiasis. This is common (see also acute complications, pages 186 to 187) and generally affects the vulva, perineum and areas of intertrigo.

Acanthosis nigricans. This condition may be seen in obese diabetics, particularly those with insulin resistance. The dusky, pigmented and hyperkeratotic lesions affect the axillae, groins and skin folds around the neck resembling true acanthosis nigricans (**815** and **816**), but in the diabetic they are benign.

815

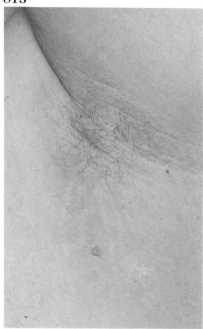

816

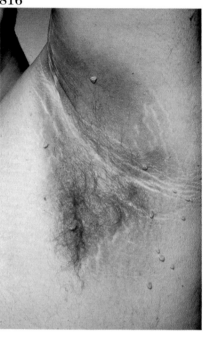

817

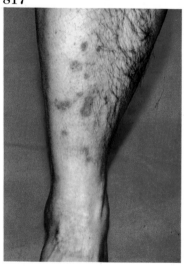

Diabetic dermopathy. The so-called 'spotted leg' consists of pigmented pretibial patches (**817**). These are small pigmented macules or oval pigmented scars in the anterior tibial regions probably resulting from local trauma.

Necrobiosis lipoidica. These are asymptomatic lesions involving the leg and are not confined to diabetics. They consist of papules (**818** to **821**) later enlarging to large plaques and these may resemble localised scleroderma (**822** and **823**). The lesions may ulcerate at a late stage (**824**) and subsequently fibrosis and involution may occur.

818

819

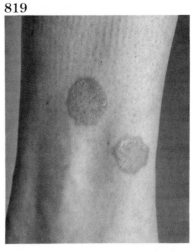

820

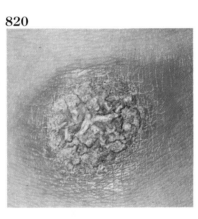

821

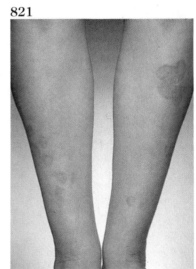

822

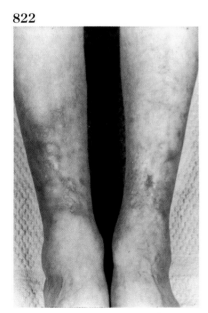

823

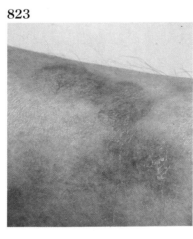

824

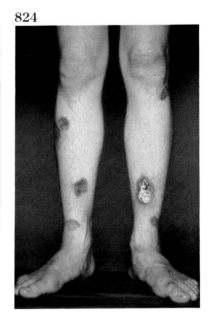

825

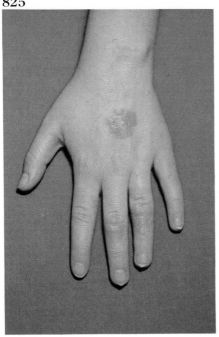

Granuloma annulare. These lesions consist of pale or flesh-coloured papules on the backs of the hands or fingers (**825** and **826**).

826

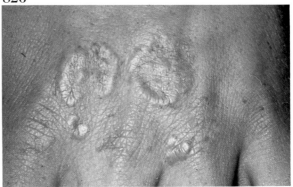

Subcutaneous lipid deposits. Xanthelasma is common in diabetes (**827**). Xanthomata are characteristically found over the tendons and the extensor surfaces of the joints. They are particularly common over the patellar and Achilles tendons (**828**), the elbows (**829** to **831**) and the metacarpophalangeal joints (**832**). Eruptive xanthomas are most commonly found over the buttocks (**833** and **834**).

827

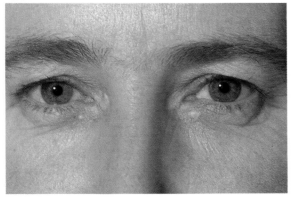

828

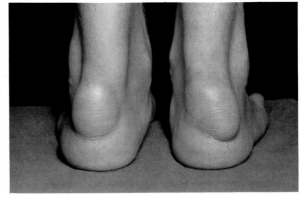

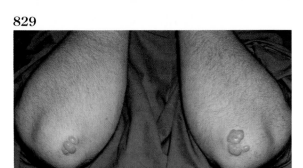

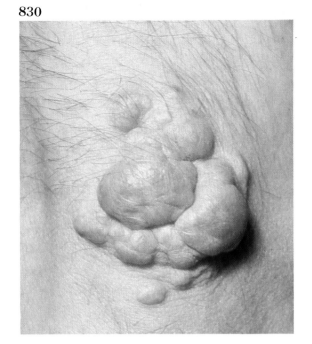

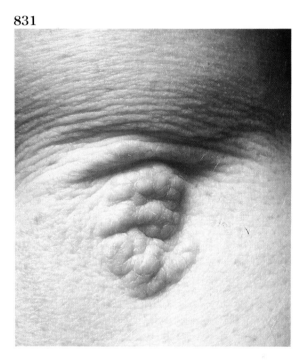

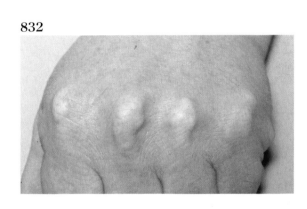

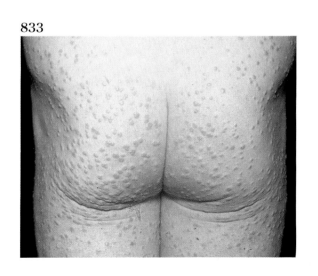

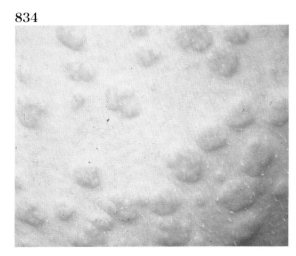

Xanthoma diabeticorum. These lesions are yellowish papules or nodules (**835** and **836**) that occur on the skin of hyperlipaemic diabetics, and consist of lipid-loaded histiocytes.

835

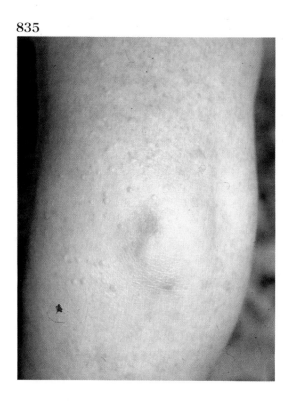

836

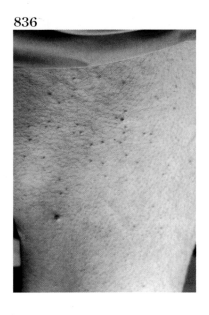

837

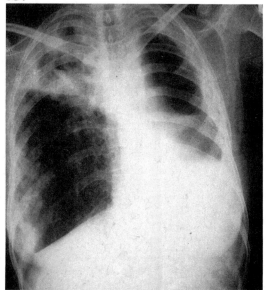

Chronic infections

Tuberculosis is common in diabetics. Investigation of unexplained weight loss, cough or fever should always include a chest radiograph. **837** shows a tuberculous lesion at the right apex and a left pleural effusion in a diabetic. Chronic urinary infections may lead to chronic renal failure. Other infections seen in diabetics include mucormycosis, necrotising fasciitis and malignant otitis externa.

Diabetic foot disease and osteopathy

Foot lesions are common in diabetics. Inspection of the feet should always be a part of the routine examination. Infections between the toes, paronychiae and chronic ulcers may lead to extensive cellulitis and gangrene (**838**). Atherosclerosis, neuropathy — autonomic and sensory, microangiopathy, infection and general debility may all contribute to the foot lesions of the diabetic. Amputation is an all too frequent sequel. Radiological changes in the feet are common and consist of arterial calcification and osteopathy — diffuse or localised osteoporosis with juxta-articular bone defects in the phalanges and the metatarsals. Later osteolysis of the bone ends (**839**) and destruction of entire bones may occur.

838

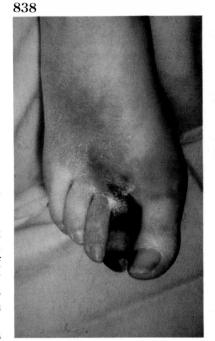

839

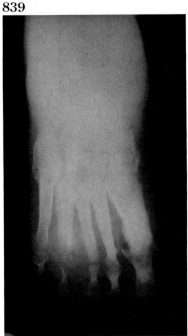

Diabetic hand syndrome

This syndrome generally occurs in insulin-dependent diabetics with peripheral neuropathy. The characteristic features are joint contractures and a waxy skin. The inability to approximate the palmar surfaces (the prayer sign) demonstrates the limited movement of all the joints (**840** and **841**).

840

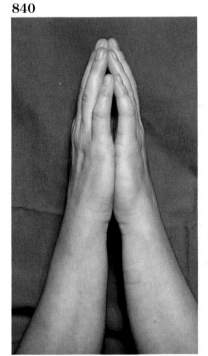

841

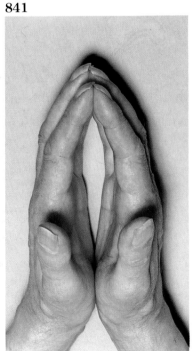

842

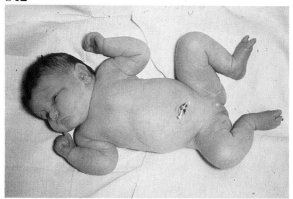

Diabetes and the fetus and neonate

Congenital malformations are more common in infants born to diabetic mothers, particularly if diabetic control has been poor in pregnancy. The lesions are of the same type as those seen in non-diabetic mothers, although multiple abnormalities are seen more frequently. Poor fetal growth and macrosomia (**842**) at term are also common in diabetic pregnancies, especially if metabolic control has been poor.

843

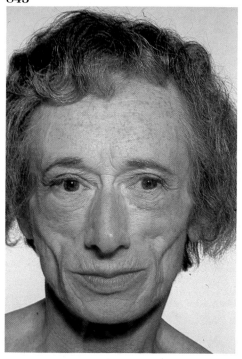

Rare diabetic syndromes

Lipoatrophic diabetes

This rare syndrome consists of non-ketotic insulin resistance, generalised atrophy of adipose tissue (shown here in the face — **843**), severe hyperlipaemia with subcutaneous xanthomatosis and hepatosplenomegaly. Acanthosis nigricans is associated with one form of the condition.

844

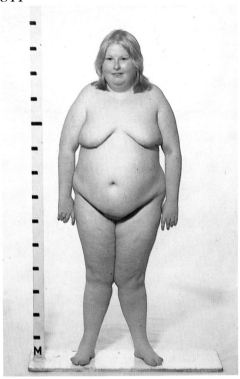

Prader–Willi syndrome

Diabetes mellitus is a frequent complication of the massive food intake characteristic of this condition. The clinical features are gross obesity, small hands and small genitalia (**844** to **847**).

845

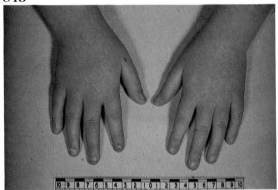

846

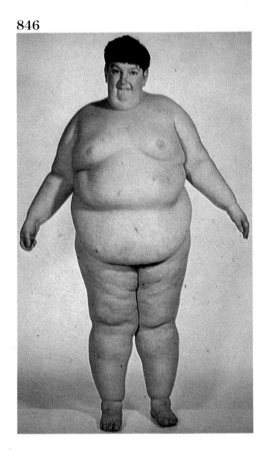

847

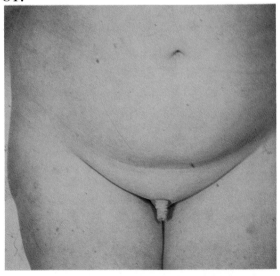

DIDMOAD syndrome

This is a rare familial condition consisting of a variety of combinations of diabetes insipidus (DI), diabetes mellitus (DM), optic atrophy (OA) and deafness (D).

Chapter 8
Pancreatic and gastrointestinal hormones and the syndromes of multiple endocrine neoplasia

Introduction

Pancreatic hormones

The endocrine cells of the pancreas are aggregated in the islets of Langerhans. Specific cells secreting insulin, glucagon, gastrin, vasoactive intestinal peptide (VIP), somatostatin and pancreatic polypeptide have all been identified. These cells form part of the APUD (amine, precursor uptake and decarboxylation) system. Clinical syndromes caused by tumours of the specific cell types can be recognised, and these tumours may secrete more than one regulatory peptide and occasionally hormones which are normally secreted at other sites (e.g. ACTH).

Gut hormones

The gastrointestinal tract contains the largest mass of endocrine cells in the body. They are widely dispersed throughout the mucosa and play a major role in regulating digestion, absorption and motility in the gut in addition to influencing bile flow, pancreatic function and regional blood flow. The major hormones of the gastrointestinal tract are:

- Gastrin — which occurs in a number of different molecular forms
- Cholecystokinin (CCK) — which also occurs in a number of forms, but the terminal octapeptide contains all the biological activity
- Vasoactive intestinal polypeptide (VIP)

- Somatostatin
- Enteroglucagon
- Secretin
- Gastric inhibitory peptide
- Motilin
- Substance P
- Neurotensin
- Pancreatic polypeptide
- Enkephalin and the endorphins
- Bombesin
- Miscellaneous other peptides

Tumours secreting gastrin, VIP, somatostatin and enteroglucagon have been described. The plasma concentrations of the other gut hormones may be secondarily increased or decreased in a number of gastrointestinal disorders. These hormones may also be secreted by other tumours of endocrine and non-endocrine origin.

Multiple endocrine neoplasia (MEN)

There are three well-documented syndromes of MEN — types I, IIa and IIb — in which there is a tendency to form tumours from a number of peptide hormone producing cells at anatomically remote sites. These may be inherited as autosomal dominants or occur sporadically.

848

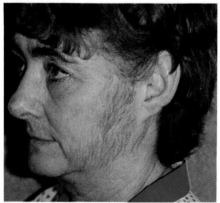

Pancreatic endocrine tumours

Insulinoma

These tumours cause hypoglycaemia, which can present in a variety of guises. It is important to differentiate hypoglycaemia caused by an islet cell tumour from factitious hypoglycaemia resulting from self-administration of insulin. Treatment of islet cell tumours with diazoxide can lead to hirsutism (**848**). Islet cell tumours may be associated with other endocrine tumours in MEN type I.

Zollinger–Ellison syndrome

Zollinger–Ellison syndrome consists of gastric hypersecretion and intractable peptic ulceration resulting from a gastrin-secreting tumour of the pancreas (85 per cent), or more rarely the duodenum (14 per cent) or stomach (1 per cent). The major clinical features are symptoms of peptic ulceration, vomiting, frequent haematemeses and diarrhoea. Radiological examination shows coarse and hypertrophied gastric mucosa (**849**). Basal acid secretion is at a very high level, and further stimulation produces very little further response as the gastric cells are already under maximum drive from the gastrin secreted by the tumour. Plasma gastrin levels are very high (greater than 150 pg/ml) but this alone is not diagnostic as high levels are also seen in pernicious anaemia. Secretion of a range of other peptide hormones (pancreatic polypeptide, somatostatin, insulin and ACTH) by gastrin-secreting tumours is common. Approximately one-third of cases occur as part of MEN type I. Some of the tumours are malignant.

Verner–Morrison syndrome and VIPomas

Verner–Morrison syndrome consists of chronic, profuse, watery diarrhoea leading to dehydration and hypokalaemia, accompanied by hypoglycaemia, hypochlorhydria and attacks of flushing (**850**). Such flushing needs to be distinguished from the much commoner menopausal flushing (**851** and **852**). Patients also tend to suffer from colicky abdominal pain, hypotension and some are hypercalcaemic. The pancreatic tumours in these patients contain large amounts of VIP (and frequently pancreatic polypeptide) and plasma levels are substantially elevated. The tumour can sometimes be demonstrated by angiography (**853**).

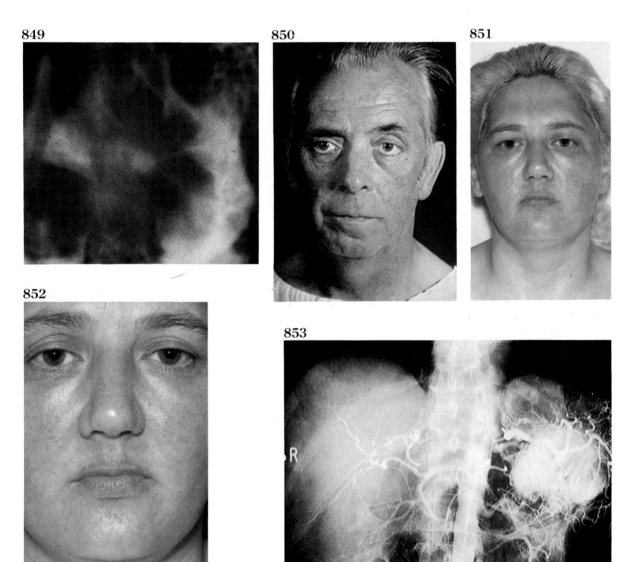

849

850

851

852

853

Glucagonoma

These pancreatic tumours are usually malignant and present with characteristic clinical features. A skin rash is often widespread. Lesions which start as erythematous areas become raised with superficial central blistering and rupture to leave crusts or weeping in areas exposed to friction (**854** to **858**). The lesions tend to heal in the centre while the edges spread with a red, crusting, well-defined margin and an annular outline. Healing is associated with increased pigmentation. Milder rashes may be seen in some patients (**859** and **860**). The rash can be produced by the administration of glucagon (**861** — given here to a patient with intractable hypogly-caemia). Patients also lose weight, are usually mildly diabetic (without ketoacidosis), frequently develop psychiatric disturbances and many suffer from major thromboembolic episodes. Plasma glucagon levels are very high (greater than 300 pmol/l). Accurate localisation of tumours may be achieved by angiography or by selective blood sampling after transhepatic catheterisation. Pancreatic endocrine tumours may change type — the patient illustrated in **859** had previously been successfully treated for a VIPoma. **862** and **863** show angiograms from the same patient before and after successful treatment of a hepatic secondary by embolisation.

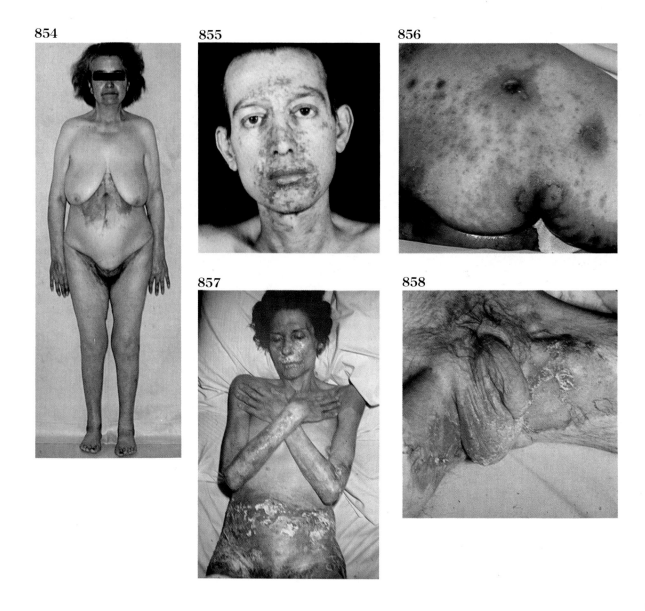

854

855

856

857

858

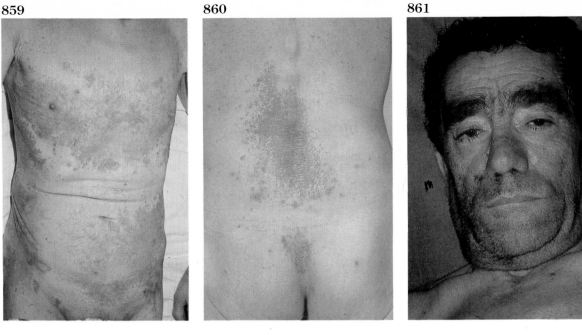

859   860   861

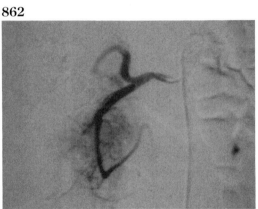

862

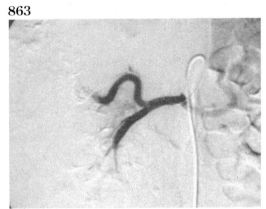

863

Somatostatinoma

Approximately twenty patients have been described with somatostatinomas. Most (80 per cent) are malignant and are located in the pancreas, although they may occur in the duodenum or jejunum or occasionally outside the gastrointestinal tract. Most tumours have been found in patients with mild diabetes and gallbladder disease, the patients are usually mildly anaemic and show some weight loss. The tumours are generally found accidentally, because of the non-specific nature of the symptoms. Somatostatinomas may present as a result of hypersecretion of another hormone — e.g. insulin or ACTH.

Pancreatic polypeptide producing tumours — PPomas

Pancreatic polypeptide (PP) levels are often found to be raised in patients with endocrine pancreatic tumours of all types — pure PPomas, VIPomas, glucagonomas, gastrinomas and insulinomas.

Miscellaneous

A range of other hormones may be secreted by tumours of the endocrine pancreas. These include growth hormone releasing hormone (GHRH), neurotensin and ACTH. Non-secretory tumours may also occur.

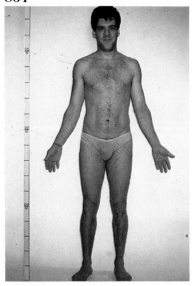

Endocrine tumours of the gastrointestinal tract

Endocrine tumours of the gastrointestinal tract are very much less common than those of the pancreas. Gastrinomas and somatostatinomas are occasionally located in the stomach, duodenum or jejunum as noted above. The clinical features are identical to those seen in patients with similar tumours arising in the pancreas. Secondary changes in the levels of the gut hormones may be seen in a number of gastrointestinal and metabolic disorders.

Multiple endocrine neoplasia (MEN)

Multiple endocrine neoplasia may occur in families, inherited as an autosomal dominant, or it may occur sporadically. Three syndromes have been described — MEN types I, IIa and IIb.

MEN type I

865

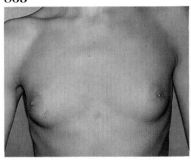

The pattern of lesions in MEN I is shown in Table 7. The finding of one of these lesions should lead to a search for the others and also to investigation of first degree relatives.

866

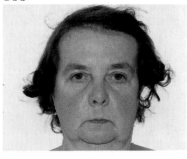

Table 7. Pattern of lesions in MEN type I.

Gland	Hormones	Disease
Pituitary	Growth hormone	Acromegaly (**864**)
	Prolactin	Amenorrhoea, galactorrhoea (**865**), impotence
	Corticotrophin	Cushing's disease (**866**)
	Non-secretory	Hypopituitarism (**867**)
Parathyroid	Parathormone	Hyperparathyroidism
Thyroid	Thyroid hormones	Toxic adenoma
	Non-secretory	Thyroid nodule
Adrenal cortex	Adrenal androgens	Hirsutism and amenorrhoea
	Cortisol	Cushing's syndrome
Pancreas	Insulin	Hypoglycaemia
	Glucagon	Rash, glossitis, diabetes
	Gastrin	Zollinger–Ellison syndrome

867

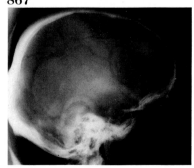

MEN types IIa and IIb

The pathological pattern of the MEN II syndromes is quite distinct from that of MEN I. It is very rare for there to be any overlap either in a patient or the family between these two major categories of multiple endocrine neoplasia. The pattern of lesions in MEN IIa is shown in Table 8.

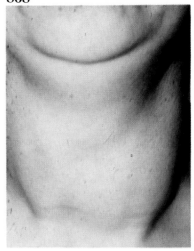

Table 8.   Pattern of lesions in MEN type IIa.

Gland	Hormones	Disease
Thyroid (C cells)	Calcitonin	Medullary carcinoma of the thyroid (**868**)
Adrenal medulla	Adrenaline, nor-adrenaline, dopamine	Phaeochromocytoma

Ectopic production of other substances — e.g. corticotrophin and serotinin — may also occur in medullary carcinoma of the thyroid.

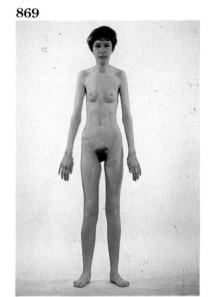

MEN IIb varies from IIa in a number of ways. This syndrome, although it may be familial, is more likely to occur sporadically. It consists of medullary carcinoma of the thyroid associated with a number of somatic abnormalities (**869**) and occasionally phaeochromocytoma or parathyroid lesions. This syndrome and the somatic abnormalities are described more fully on page 117.

Chapter 9
Calcium, the parathyroids and metabolic bone disease

Introduction

The calcium content of the adult human body amounts to about 25 moles, of which about 99 per cent is in the skeleton. The daily dietary intake of calcium varies widely. Calcium absorption takes place by one of two processes — passive or active. The major factor controlling calcium absorption is vitamin D. The normal range for total plasma calcium is about 2.2 to 2.6 mmol/l, and just under one-half of this is present as free calcium ions. The major humoral factors involved in calcium homeostasis are parathyroid hormone (PTH) and vitamin D. No clear physiological role has been identified for calcitonin in man.

PTH is an 84 amino-acid polypeptide which acts on specific receptors on the plasma membrane of target cells. Its primary function is to regulate ionised calcium concentration in body fluids and its principal sites of action are the kidney and bone. PTH has only an indirect influence on intestinal absorption of calcium by stimulating renal synthesis of 1,25 dihydroxy-cholecalciferol, the main active metabolite of vitamin D. The most potent stimulus to PTH secretion is hypocalcaemia, and the reciprocal relationship which exists between PTH and plasma calcium results from a direct feedback mechanism.

The active forms of vitamin D are derived from ergocalciferol (D2) which is available only from the diet, and cholecalciferol (D3) which is synthesised in the skin and is also available in some foods. The major active metabolite is 1,25 dihydroxycholecalciferol which has its primary action on the intestine, stimulating calcium and phosphate absorption. It also stimulates renal tubular reabsorption of calcium and phosphate and mobilises these elements from bone.

Diseases of the parathyroids

Hyperparathyroidism

Hyperparathyroidism may be primary, secondary or tertiary.

Primary hyperparathyroidism

Primary hyperparathyroidism may result from adenoma (about 85 per cent), hyperplasia (about 12 per cent) or carcinoma (about 3 per cent). Adenomas and hyperplasia may occur as part of the syndromes of multiple endocrine neoplasia (MEN). In MEN type I hyperparathyroidism may be associated with adenomas of the pituitary, pancreas, adrenal and possibly the thyroid. In MEN II hyperparathyroidism is associated with medullary carcinoma or C cell hyperplasia of the thyroid and phaeochromocytoma or hyperplasia of the adrenal medulla.

Clinical features of hyperparathyroidism (870). These fall naturally into four categories:

- Symptoms caused by hypercalcaemia:
Anorexia, nausea and vomiting
Constipation
Weight loss
Muscle weakness (proximal myopathy)
Polyuria and polydipsia (primary polyuria)
Psychiatric disturbances
Pruritus

- Features caused by metastatic calcification:
Conjunctival deposits
Corneal deposits (band keratopathy)
Renal calculi
Nephrocalcinosis
Renal failure
Pseudo-gout
Pancreatitis

- Features caused by bone disease:
Bone pain
Skeletal deformities
Pathological fractures
Bone tumours (osteoclastomas)

- Features caused by associated pathology:
Hypertension
Peptic ulcer
Zollinger–Ellison syndrome
Hyperuricaemia leading to true gout
Neonatal tetany (from maternal hyperparathyroidism)
Features caused by other components of MEN I or II

It should be stressed, however, that with the improvement in diagnostic techniques which has taken place in recent years, the diagnosis is now frequently made when the patient is asymptomatic or exhibiting only the non-specific symptoms of hypercalcaemia.

870

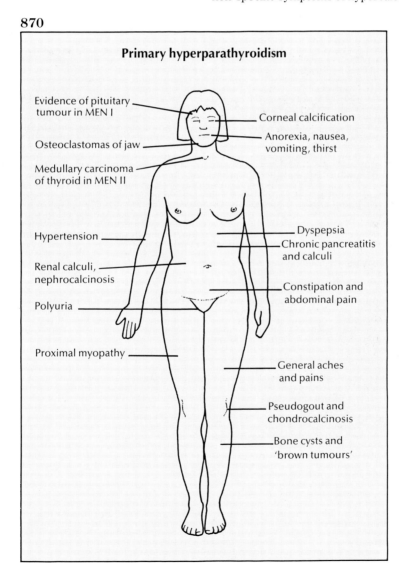

Primary hyperparathyroidism

- Evidence of pituitary tumour in MEN I
- Osteoclastomas of jaw
- Medullary carcinoma of thyroid in MEN II
- Hypertension
- Renal calculi, nephrocalcinosis
- Polyuria
- Proximal myopathy
- Corneal calcification
- Anorexia, nausea, vomiting, thirst
- Dyspepsia
- Chronic pancreatitis and calculi
- Constipation and abdominal pain
- General aches and pains
- Pseudogout and chondrocalcinosis
- Bone cysts and 'brown tumours'

Clinical features caused by metastatic calcification. Hypercalcaemia may lead to ectopic calcification in the conjunctiva or in the lateral margins of the cornea — band keratopathy (**871** and **872**). This must be distinguished from arcus, which first develops at the upper and lower limbi of the cornea and eventually becomes circumferential (**873**).

Nephrocalcinosis (**874**) and renal stone formation (**875**) are common complications of primary hyperparathyroidism and because the stones contain calcium they are radio-opaque. Renal failure may result.

It is important from a diagnostic and therapeutic point of view to distinguish between renal failure caused by primary hyperparathyroidism and secondary hyperparathyroidism caused by renal failure.

Calcification in joint cartilages is found in some cases, producing chondrocalcinosis. This is most frequently seen in the knees (**876** and **877**) and may be complicated by pseudo-gout.

Acute, subacute or chronic pancreatitis may be associated with pancreatic calculi or calcification (**878**).

871

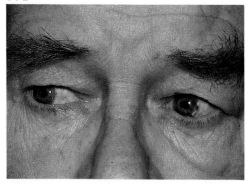

872

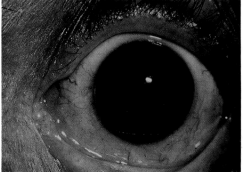

873

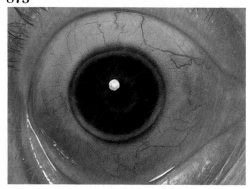

874

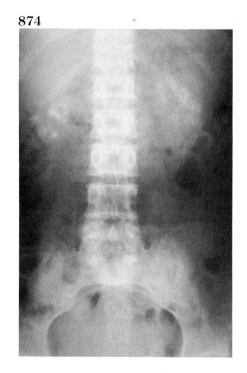

875

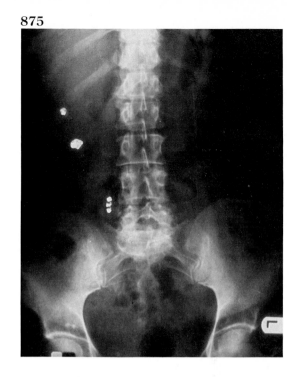

876

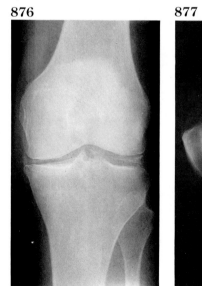

877

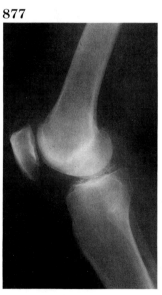

878

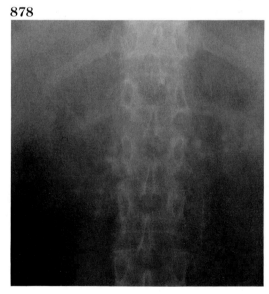

Clinical features caused by bone disease. Osteitis fibrosa may cause general aches and pains, sometimes severe bone pain, tenderness and even fractures and deformities. The characteristic radiological signs are osteopenia and subperiosteal erosions of the phalanges and terminal digital tufts (**879** and **880**). The erosions are usually seen most clearly on the radial aspects of the middle phalanges and also in the outer third of the clavicle. Bone cysts may be solitary (**881**) or multiple (**882**). The skull may also show a granular or mottled appearance like ground glass, and sometimes cystic areas are apparent (**883** and **884**). Loss of the lamina dura around the teeth (**885**) may be seen by comparison with the normal jaw (**886**). Rarely, cysts or osteoclastomas of the jaw (**887**) or long bones (**888**) may be presenting features. Osteoporosis may be increased.

879

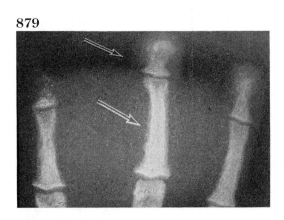

880

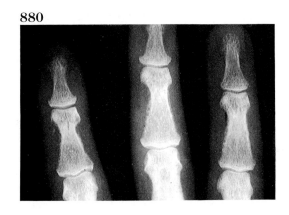

881

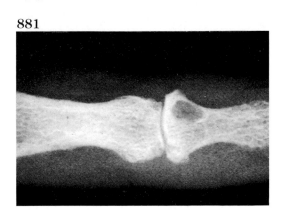

882

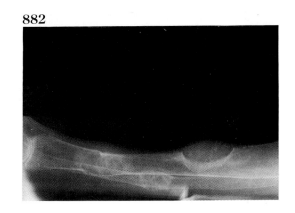

883

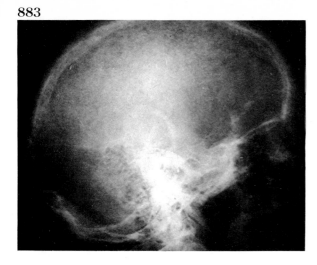

884

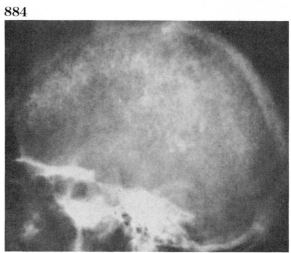

885

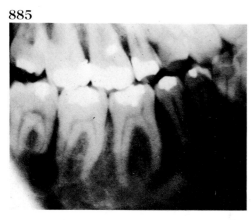

886

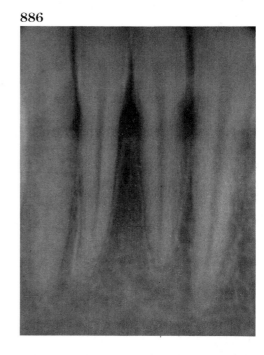

887

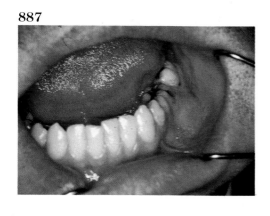

888

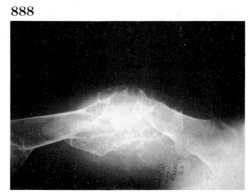

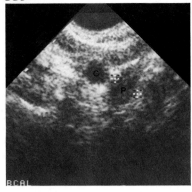

889

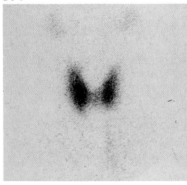

890

Diagnosis of primary hyperparathyroidism. Two major steps are involved. The first is to confirm the diagnosis and to distinguish between primary hyperparathyroidism and other causes of hypercalcaemia, and the second is to localise the tumour or tumours — particularly in patients who have previously been exposed to an unsuccessful neck exploration. The localisation of parathyroid tumours poses many problems. None of the methods currently available is entirely satisfactory and no technique is particularly reliable for identifying small tumours. The methods in current use include radionuclide scanning using either selenomethionine or ^{201}thallium/^{99m}technetium subtraction scanning, computerised axial tomography, arteriography and selective venous catheterisation and sampling for parathyroid hormone levels. The latter two techniques are rarely used now: arteriography is also associated with a considerable morbidity. **889** shows a transverse ultrasound scan of a parathyroid adenoma (P = parathyroid adenoma, C = common carotid artery). **890** to **892** demonstrate a parathyroid adenoma by the thallium/technetium subtraction technique (**890** shows the technetium image of the thyroid, **891** the thallium image of the thyroid and parathyroids, and **892** the subtracted image with abnormal activity just below the right lower pole of the thyroid). **893** shows a contrast-enhanced CT scan with adenoma arrowed (C = common carotid artery, S = strap muscles).

The cardinal biochemical features of primary hyperparathyroidism are an elevated fasting plasma calcium in the presence of a raised or normal (i.e. inappropriately high) parathyroid hormone concentration. Other biochemical abnormalities reflecting the perturbation of calcium and phosphate homeostasis are of secondary importance for diagnostic purposes.

891

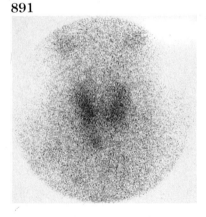

892

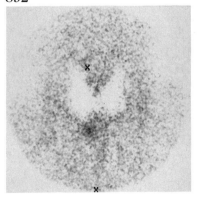

893

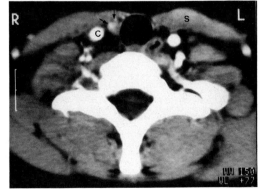

Other important causes of hypercalcaemia include:

a) *Sarcoidosis*, in which lupus-like skin infiltration (**894** and **895**), nail changes (**896**) and cystic bone lesions (**897** and **898**) may be present. **899** shows a chest radiograph with typical hilar lymphadenopathy.

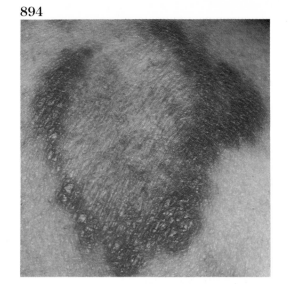
894

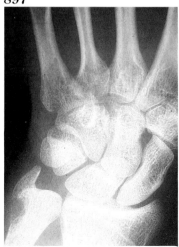
895

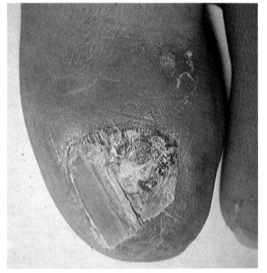
896

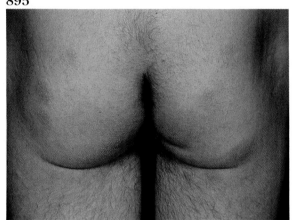
897

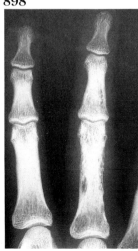
898

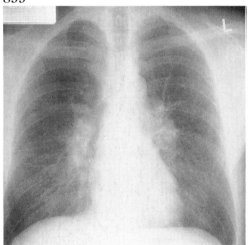
899

900

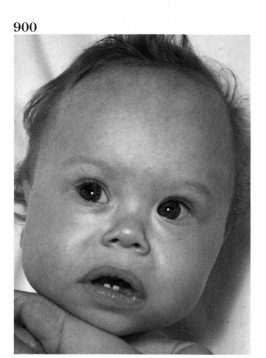

b) *Vitamin D intoxication* or sensitivity leading to 'idiopathic hypercalcaemia' of infancy leading to the characteristic elfin appearance (**900**).

c) *Bone diseases* — including osteolytic secondary deposits which may be demonstrated radiologically (**901** and **902**) or by bone scanning (**903**), myelomatosis (**904** and **905**), Paget's disease of bone (**906** and **907**) and rarely osteoporosis (**908**) after immobilisation. The clinical and radiological features of these disorders may occasionally be mistaken for hyperparathyroidism.

901

902

903

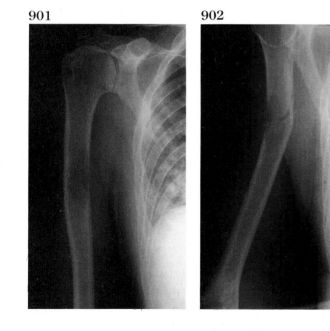

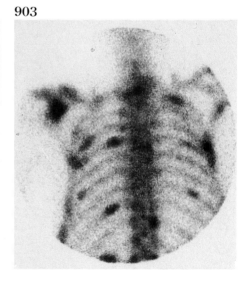

904

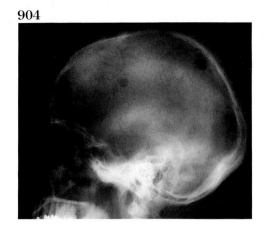

905

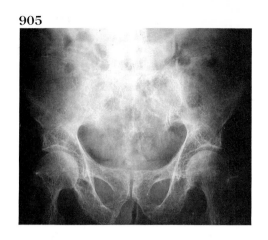

906

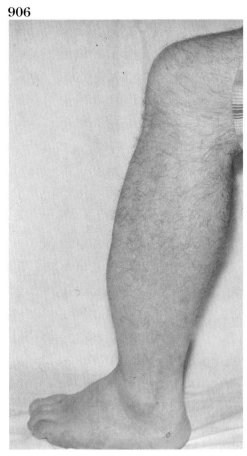

907

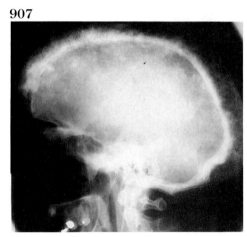

908

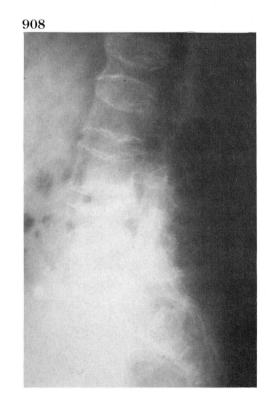

Secondary hyperparathyroidism

Secondary hyperparathyroidism results from hypocalcaemia leading to hyperplasia of all four parathyroids. The commonest cause is chronic renal failure. The clinical features of renal failure are generally apparent. **909** shows a patient with a typically uraemic appearance. **910** shows secondary hyperparathyroidism in chronic renal failure. Osteosclerosis may also be present (**911** and **912**). Secondary hyperparathyroidism may also be associated with vitamin D deficiency in rickets and osteomalacia (**913** shows a 'rugger jersey' spine — see also below). The plasma calcium may be low or normal and the plasma phosphate is variable but is frequently elevated in chronic renal failure. The parathyroid hormone level is raised. It should be remembered that primary and secondary hyperparathyroidism may coexist in patients with chronic renal failure and this may complicate the biochemical picture.

909

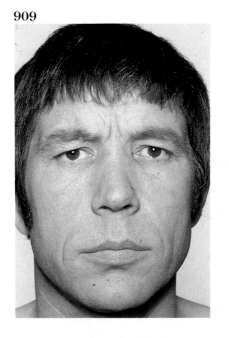

910

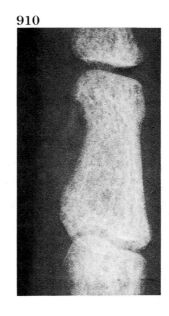

Tertiary hyperparathyroidism

The term tertiary hyperparathyroidism is used to describe patients who develop parathyroid adenomas causing hypercalcaemia on a background of reactive or secondary hyperplasia.

911

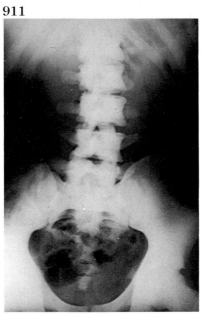

912

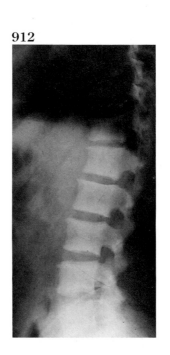

913

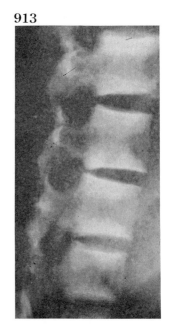

Hypoparathyroidism

The clinical features of hypoparathyroidism may result from a failure of parathyroid hormone secretion or from failure of its action at tissue level (pseudohypoparathyroidism). The causes of failure of parathyroid hormone secretion are:

- Neonatal hypoparathyroidism. This may occur transiently a) in children born to mothers with hyperparathyroidism, b) precipitated by a high phosphate diet or c) associated with hypoglycaemia — or permanently, caused by congenital absence of the parathyroids.
- Post-surgical hypoparathyroidism
- Idiopathic hypoparathyroidism
- DiGeorge syndrome
- MEDAC syndrome

The major clinical features of hypoparathyroidism are shown in **914**. Many of these result from hypocalcaemia. They include tetany, which is a complex of symptoms and signs including carpopedal spasm (**915** and **916**), muscle cramps, paraesthesiae of the hands, feet and circumoral region and neuromuscular irritability, which may be demonstrated by tapping the facial nerve in front of the ear causing twitching of the facial muscles — Chvostek's sign. In severe tetanic attacks there is hyperreflexia and, in children, laryngeal stridor and convulsions. Epilepsy, mental deterioration and psychological disturbances may result from prolonged hypocalcaemia.

914

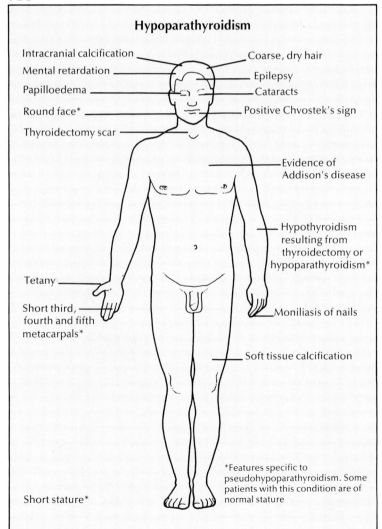

Hypoparathyroidism

Intracranial calcification
Mental retardation
Papilloedema
Round face*
Thyroidectomy scar

Coarse, dry hair
Epilepsy
Cataracts
Positive Chvostek's sign

Evidence of Addison's disease

Hypothyroidism resulting from thyroidectomy or hypoparathyroidism*

Tetany

Short third, fourth and fifth metacarpals*

Moniliasis of nails

Soft tissue calcification

*Features specific to pseudohypoparathyroidism. Some patients with this condition are of normal stature

Short stature*

915

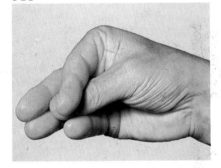

916

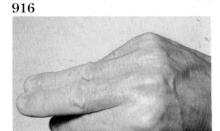

917

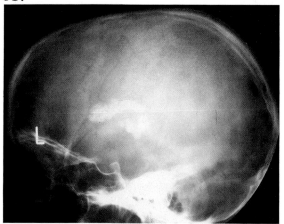

Intracranial sequelae of hypoparathyroidism include raised intracranial pressure, papilloedema and symmetrical, bilateral calcification of the basal ganglia, which may be seen radiologically (**917** and **918**) or on CT scan (**919**).

918

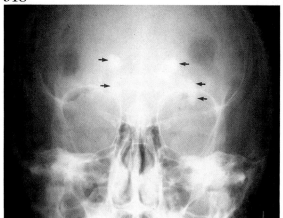

919

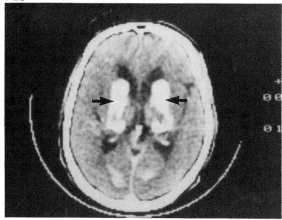

920

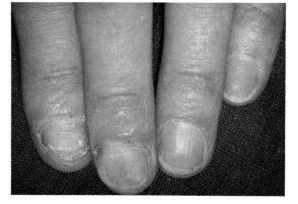

Cataracts may result from long-standing hypocalcaemia from any cause. The skin and hair may be coarse and dry and the nails brittle and deformed. Candidiasis of the skin and nails is often resistant to therapy (**920**).

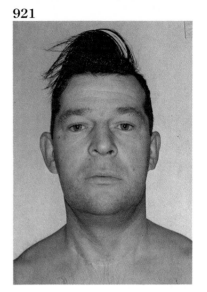

921

Hypoparathyroidism most commonly occurs **post-surgically** and is a potentially dangerous complication of neck surgery, usually occurring after partial or total thyroidectomy (**921** — note scar on neck).

Failure to secrete parathyroid hormone may be familial and is sometimes associated with vitiligo (**922**) or idiopathic (autoimmune) Addison's disease (**923**). DiGeorge syndrome is characterised by congenital absence of the parathyroids and the thymus, leading to depression of cell-mediated immune responses, which results in recurrent and severe infections. There are often associated developmental abnormalities and these include hypertelorism, low-set ears, micrognathia and anomalies of the aorta and great vessels. MEDAC syndrome is the association of multiple endocrine deficiency, autoimmunity and candidiasis. The syndrome is characterised by reduced function of the parathyroids and the adrenals with organ-specific autoantibodies and candidiasis. Pernicious anaemia, thyroiditis, premature ovarian failure and hepatitis may also occur.

922

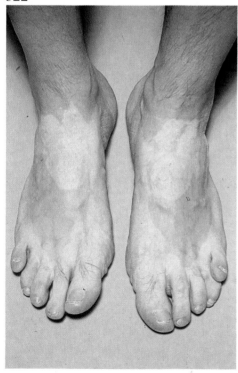

923

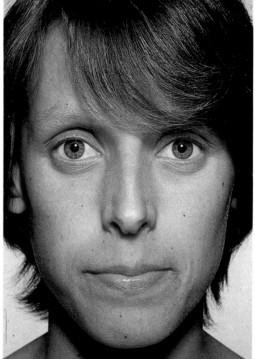

Pseudohypoparathyroidism

Failure of parathyroid hormone action results in the syndrome of pseudohypoparathyroidism, a familial condition which occurs approximately twice as frequently in females as in males. The syndrome is characterised by mental retardation, short stature (**924**), a round face and short neck (**925**), abnormal teeth (**926**), and shortness of the third, fourth and fifth metacarpals (**927** and **928**, compared in **929** with the normal on the right). Radiographs of the hands and feet (**930** to **932**) demonstrate the short metacarpals and metatarsals respectively. There is an increased incidence of hypothyroidism and diabetes mellitus. The plasma calcium is low as in hypoparathyroidism, but the parathyroid hormone levels are raised — indicating a failure of peripheral tissue response. The term pseudo-pseudohypoparathyroidism is used to refer to patients with the somatic abnormalities but without the biochemical features of pseudohypoparathyroidism.

924

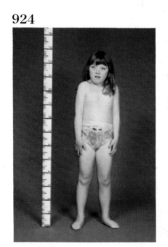

925

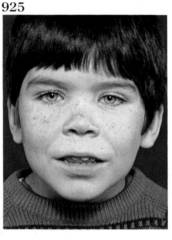

926

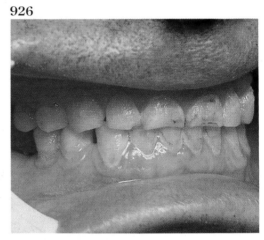

927

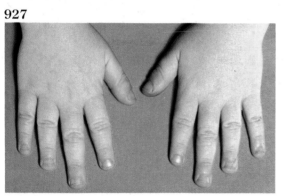

928

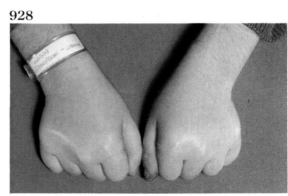

929

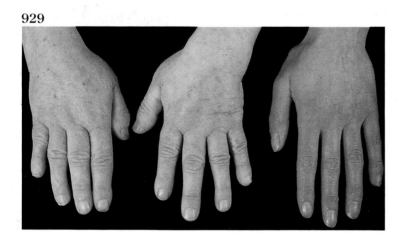

930

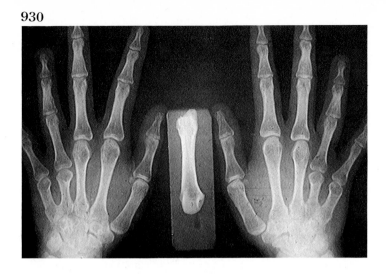

931

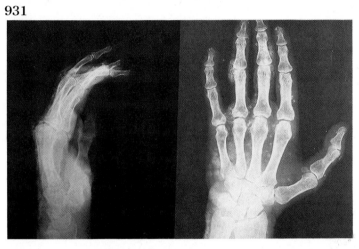

932

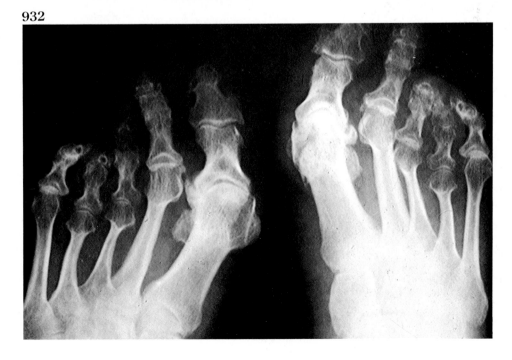

Metabolic bone disease

Rickets and osteomalacia

Rickets and osteomalacia result from defective mineralisation, generally caused by deficiency of vitamin D. Rickets is the consequence of vitamin D deficiency in childhood, and osteomalacia that in adult life. The major causes are:

1. Dietary deficiency of vitamin D

2. Malabsorption of vitamin D (resulting from gastrectomy, small intestinal disease or chronic liver disease)

3. Chronic renal failure

4. Renal tubular acidosis

5. Hypophosphataemia

6. Disorders of vitamin D metabolism

7. Factors which interfere with mineralisation (e.g. aluminium, diphosphonates, fluorides)

Skeletal deformities are common in rickets. Growth is often retarded and dentition is delayed. Children frequently develop bow legs or knock knees (**933** to **935**) and thickening of the wrists (**936**), prominence of the costochondral junction and frontal bossing may be seen. Hypotonia and myopathy are common. The most characteristic feature of osteomalacia is bone pain and tenderness. Pathological fractures may occur and a proximal myopathy is common.

The **radiological features of rickets** are seen early in the natural history of the disease and are pathognomonic. There is widening and cupping of the epiphyseal growth plates (**937** and **938**) and these improve after treatment (**939**). There may also be thinning of the cortical bone. The characteristic radiological changes of osteomalacia are seen relatively late in the course of the disease.

933

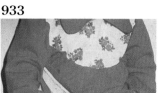
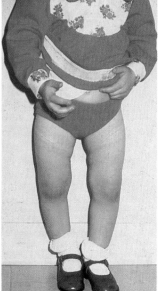

934

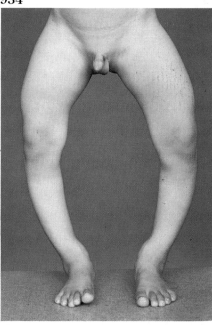

935

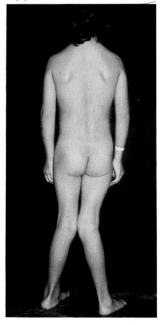

936

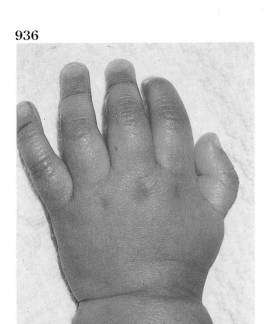

937

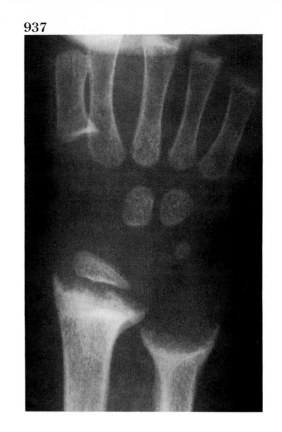

938

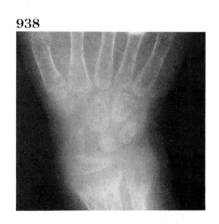

939

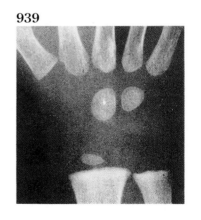

940

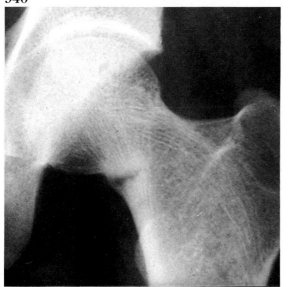

The pathognomonic radiological change in osteomalacia is the **presence of Looser's zones or pseudofractures**. These are lucent zones extending from the surface of the bone through the cortex to the trabecular bone. They are often bilateral and are most commonly seen in the femoral necks, pubic rami, ribs and the axillary borders of the scapulae (**940** to **942**). There is also a coarse trabecular pattern in the vertebrae (**943**). Reduced bone density and pathological fractures may also be seen. The characteristic biochemical changes are a reduced plasma calcium, a reduced phosphate (if renal function is normal) and an elevated alkaline phosphatase. Bone histology shows an increase in osteoid volume and osteoid seam width with a reduction in the calcification front (**944**).

941

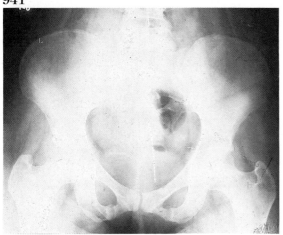

942

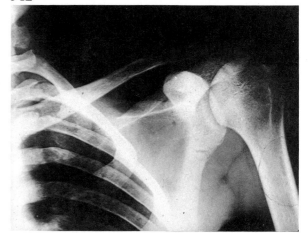

943

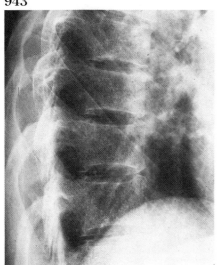

944

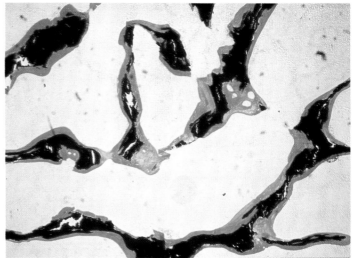

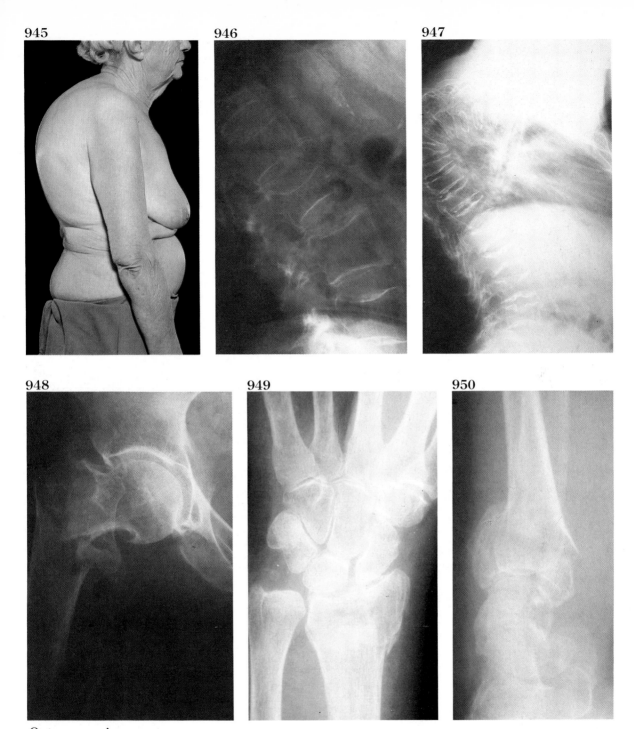

Osteoporosis

Osteoporosis is the term used to describe a reduction in bone mass. Loss of bone mass is an ineluctable consequence of advancing age and may be particularly rapid in women after the menopause. Osteoporosis may also occur as a result of some endocrine disorders (Cushing's syndrome, hyperthyroidism, hyperparathyroidism and premature ovarian failure), malabsorption syndromes, immobilisation and chronic renal failure. A reduction in bone mass is also seen in osteogenesis imperfecta, which results from specific disorders of collagen cross-linking. Osteoporosis is frequently asymptomatic. There may be loss of height as a result of vertebral compression, and this may be associated with kyphosis (**945** and **946**). Fractures are common and the most frequent of these are crush fractures of the vertebrae, fractures of the femoral neck and Colles' fracture (distal end of the radius) (**947** to **950**).

Radiological changes in osteoporosis in the absence of fractures are seen late in the disease. There is a reduction in bone density with thinning of the cortices of the long bones (**951**), and loss of trabecular pattern in the vertebrae, which may become wedge-shaped (**952**). Protrusion of the intervertebral disc into the vertebrae produces the characteristic cod-fish appearance. The plasma biochemistry is normal and bone biopsy is generally unhelpful. Osteogenesis imperfecta is characterised by abnormalities of collagen structure leading to blue sclerae (**953**), fragile bones and frequent fractures (see page 60).

951

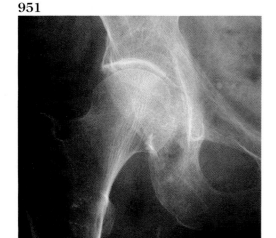

952

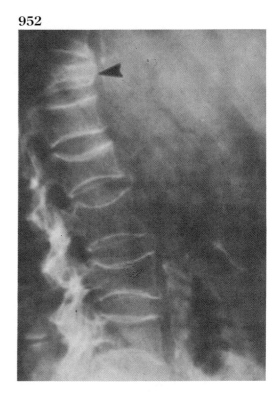

953

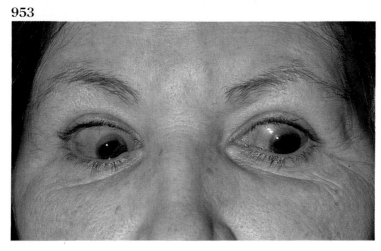

Paget's disease of bone

Paget's disease is characterised by excessive bone resorption, turnover and remodelling. The bone mass is increased but the bone is architecturally abnormal and its structural strength is diminished. The bones most frequently affected are the skull, lumbosacral vertebrae, pelvis, femora and tibiae. The most common symptom is bone pain. Deformity may occur and this is most commonly manifested as an increase in skull size and bowing of the long bones of the lower limbs (**954** and **955**). The affected bone is highly vascular and skin temperature is increased over the limb. Rarely, symptoms may occur as a result of pressure on structures in bony canals (e.g. deafness caused by auditory nerve pressure, facial nerve palsy or compression of the brain-stem or spinal cord). **956** shows a patient with severe Paget's disease affecting the skull bones with a facial palsy and deafness (note the hearing aid). Osteosarcoma is a rare complication of Paget's disease.

954

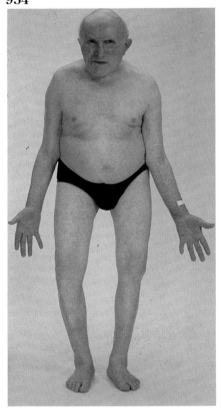

955

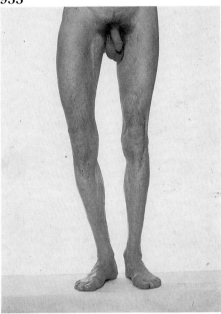

956

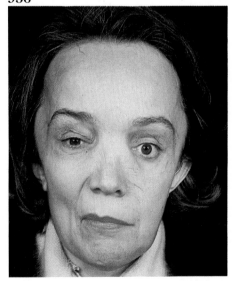

Radiologically, the bones are expanded and deformed with loss of corticomedullary definition and a coarse and abnormal trabecular pattern (**957** to **960**). The increased bone vascularity and turnover is clearly demonstrated by a bone scan (**961** and **962**). There is a striking improvement in bone morphology following treatment (**963**, before treatment on left, and after on right). Plasma calcium and phosphate levels are generally normal although prolonged immobilisation may lead to an increase in plasma calcium. The alkaline phosphatase and urinary hydroxyproline are elevated, reflecting increased osteoblastic and osteoclastic activity respectively.

957

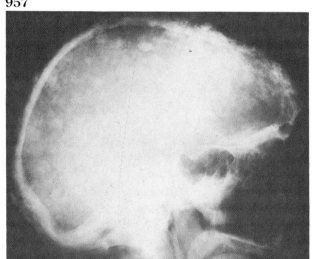

958

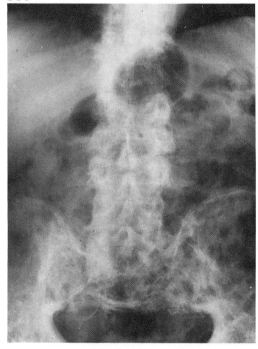

959

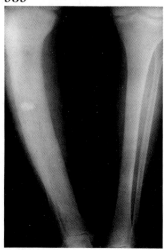

960

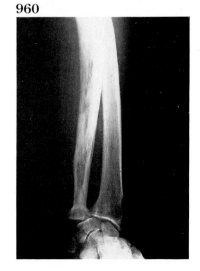

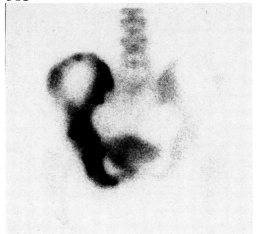

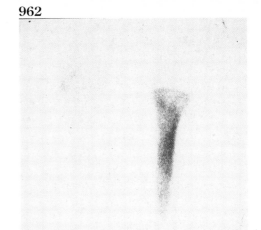

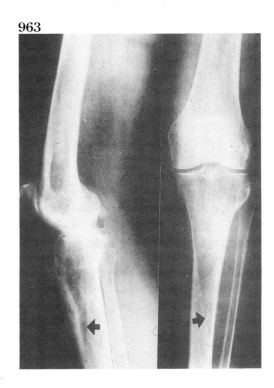

Polyostotic fibrous dysplasia (Albright's syndrome)

The bone is replaced in fibrous dysplasia by fibrous vascular tissue. The lesions may affect one bone only (monostotic) or a number of bones (polyostotic). Polyostotic fibrous dysplasia may be associated with skin pigmentation and sexual precocity (see pages 40 and 161). Associations with goitre, hyperthyroidism, acromegaly and Cushing's disease have also been reported.

Index